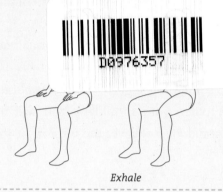

Exhale

Your chin is moving one way and your shoulders are twisting the other direction. This movement increases the stretch on the outside of your neck. As before, alternate sides and repeat four times. To deepen the stretch on the outside of your neck, stay in the twist for three breaths and then return to the start position.

Sit, breathe, and feel your neck and middle back. I am sure you can feel the results of these simple twists. You have had a nice stretch and you have increased blood, oxygen, and energy in the area of your neck and back.

* **Keep in Mind:** *Exhale* and *Twist / Inhale* and *Unwind*.

* **Cautions:** Keep neck long—neither lift nor drop the chin.

* **Other Benefits:** Increased suppleness in cervical and thoracic spine. Clearer thinking due to increased blood and energy flow to the brain.

*When twisting the spine, lower back, mid-back, or neck, as we were just doing, always twist while **exhaling** and come out of the twist while **inhaling**.*
Now, try those twists again. Do all three variations of twisting

your neck and shoulders while exhaling and emptying your breath from the bottom of your lungs with a slight contraction below the navel. When you inhale, fill from top to bottom.

When you finish, sit, breathe, and scan your body from head to toe. Notice how your neck and middle back feel.

Now let's do something slightly more complicated to open your upper body and loosen your shoulders. You will notice that when you relax your shoulders, it relieves the tension in your neck.

Your Neck, Upper Back, and Shoulders

* **Keep in Mind:** When sweeping your arms, push your fingertips away to straighten the arms and open the shoulders. Start your exhale by gently pulling in below your navel.

* **Cautions:** Do not force your arms to move farther than your shoulders will allow.

* **Other Benefits:** Increased mobility in the shoulders.

Sit forward in a chair without arms, with your feet flat on the floor (or other support) and knees wide apart, and bring your palms together in front of your chest. Keeping your elbows down, inhale, and notice that your breastbone (sternum) lifts as you inhale and open your forearms as far to your sides as you comfortably can. Do this without compressing your lower back or lifting your chin. Keep the lift at the sternum, start your exhale, then close your arms, bringing your palms back together.

YOUR NECK FIG. # 4

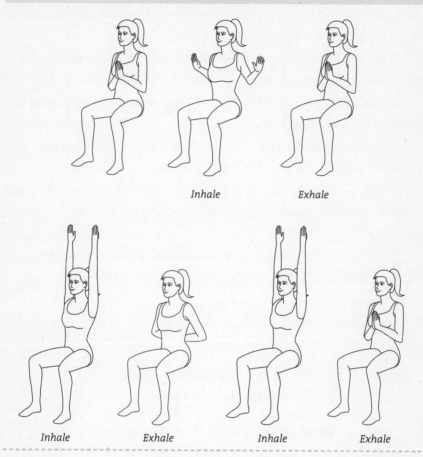

Inhale   Exhale

Inhale   Exhale   Inhale   Exhale

With your next inhale, open and extend your arms as you sweep them out to the side, and then bring them up over your head. Come to a full stop of breathing and moving. Exhale, lower your arms (this time taking your hands behind you and turning your palms so that the backs of your hands rest in the lower back area). Feel your arm bones (humerus) rotate in your shoulder as you lower your arms.

When you sweep your arms, push your fingertips away from you to lengthen and straighten your arms and to open your shoulders.

Inhale, sweep your hands up over your head, and come to a full stop. Exhale, lower your arms, and bring your palms together in front of your chest, the start position.

Repeat each of these exercises a few times, because repetition will transform the way you use your body in your daily life. In fact, the most significant musculoskeletal and neuromuscular transformation happens by repeating movements.

If these sequences feel a little awkward at first, remember that yoga will take a little practice before you get the hang of it.

When you finish, sit and breathe. See and feel the four divisions of your breath. Inhale, pause, exhale, pause. Scan your body from head to toe.

If a muscle or joint feels sore or irritated, you may have done too much. Just do a little less tomorrow, but be sure to do something.

Yoga Sutra II-46
STHIRA-SUKHAM-ASANAM

Asana (postures) must have the dual qualities
of alertness and relaxation.

The goal of Viniyoga is to create these dual qualities of alertness and relaxation by using gradual, appropriate movement. It is called *Vinyasa krama*. A sequence or Vinyasa (a series of asanas connected by breath and movement) is created in a step-by-step manner. The deeper goal of Viniyoga is to create these dual qualities of alertness and relaxation in all of life.

YOUR COMPLETE NECK SEQUENCE

* * *

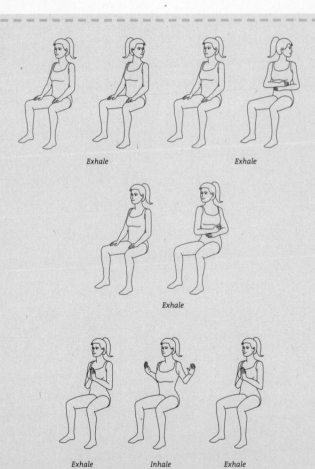

Exhale   Exhale

Exhale

Exhale   Inhale   Exhale

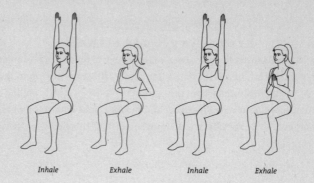

Inhale   *Exhale*   *Inhale*   *Exhale*

Tension Headache

Many "tension" headaches are caused by constriction of the muscles in the neck, shoulders, and upper back. Sweeping your arms and turning your head in proper sequence will release the tension caused by tight muscles and facilitate proper blood and energy flow up the neck to the head and brain.

I recently helped a friend in her office and was working on her computer. She uses an Apple Macintosh rather than the PC that I use at home. The standard issue keyboard and mouse that come with Macs are too small for my large hands. Also, the monitor was too high and her chair too low. After just one day, my headache told me there was a problem. We solved it by lowering the monitor, raising my chair, and getting a larger size keyboard and mouse. The lesson here is to pay attention to ergonomics and, in all cases, use the tools that fit your body. A good carpenter knows which hammer is the correct one for the job at hand. He would never use a small tack hammer to pound the large nails required to frame a house. If he did, his hand and arm would be aching in less than an hour. When working at the computer, adjust your monitor and chair height so that you are looking straight ahead at the monitor, not lifting your chin and thus compressing your cervical spine. This alone will save you a lot of soreness and pain at the end of the day and in years to come.

Disclaimer: This chapter is for **tension headaches, not migraine headaches**. The asanas shown here (that have you bend forward and put your head below your waist) will increase the blood pressure in the head and brain. This is fine for people who suffer occasionally from tension headaches. *This is not appropriate for a migraine headache. It increases the blood pressure, which will exacerbate rather than relieve the problem. If you suffer with migraine headaches, consult your physician for treatment.*

Tension Headache Relief

• Start by sitting up comfortably straight in a chair. Pay attention to your breathing. Feel the easy inhale and exhale in your nostrils. Let the top of your head float up as if there is a puppeteer's string attached that is gently lengthening your neck.

• As you exhale, consciously relax your head, your face, and your jaw. Release your tongue away from the roof of your mouth. Relax your scalp. It may take a couple of exhales to do this. Continue breathing.

• Move on and relax your shoulders. Let them drop to a comfortable position.

• Use your next exhale to relax your upper back and chest.

• Then relax your stomach and lower back. Try to do this without slouching, just relaxing. Work your way down to the soles of your feet.

• Place the palms of your hands over your closed eyes and breathe a few more breaths.

Now you are ready to begin moving your neck and shoulders. Start with the gentle neck and shoulder twists (see Your Neck on page 13). Turn your chin left and right as you exhale, returning to the center as you inhale. Turn your chin and shoulders in the same direction. Turn your chin one direction and your shoulders in the opposite direction and hold that position for four or five breaths. Don't strain. Try to feel stable and reasonably comfortable in the holding position.

While holding the twist, gently tilt your head sideways, moving your ear toward the near shoulder. This will increase the stretch of the neck muscles.

TENSION HEADACHE FIG. # 1

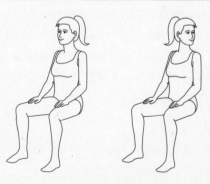

Exhale

TENSION HEADACHE FIG. # 1 (*CONTINUED*)

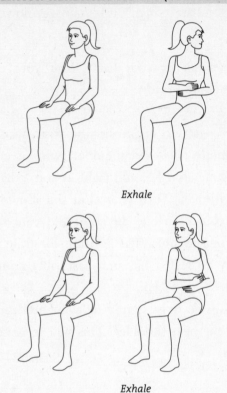

Exhale

Exhale

Next, we will combine three movements: sweeping one arm, turning the chin, and folding forward. This Vinyasa (two or more asanas connected with breath and movement) can be done sitting in a chair or kneeling on the floor. I will describe the movement for the floor.

Tension Headache

VAJRASANA (VAJRA=DIAMOND, KNEEL, SPINE)

* **Keep in Mind:** Push the tops of your feet into the floor for balance while bending forward and coming up. Push your fingertips away to straighten your arms and open your shoulders. To come up, lift your chest, not your chin.

* **Cautions:** If you can't keep your balance bending forward while kneeling, or if kneeling is uncomfortable, do this asana in a chair for awhile.

* **Other Benefits:** Lower back stretching and strengthening.

When I get down on the floor, I like to use a yoga mat. Mine is a small Navajo area rug about three feet by six feet. Some people use a foam pad. I understand there is a Gucci yoga mat available for about four hundred dollars, although a clean beach towel will do nicely. Later in the sequence you will be placing your face on the floor. As you can see, yoga can be done anywhere, but if possible find a spot that doesn't get a lot of foot traffic from shoes that are worn outside. You wouldn't want to put your face down on the floor in front of the door leading in from the garage, if you know what I mean.

If you need more padding under your knees to comfortably kneel on them, place a folded blanket or towel on top of your yoga mat. Have enough padding under your knees to be comfortable but not so much that you are wobbly. While kneeling, press the tops of your feet into the floor for balance. Place your hands, palms up, in your lower back or by your sides.

Inhale, lengthen your spine, and sweep your **right** arm up, over your head.

TENSION HEADACHE FIG. # 2

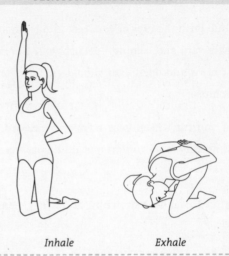

Inhale   Exhale

Start your exhale by pulling in slightly with your lower abdominal muscles. As you fold forward, bending your knees slightly, sweep your arm behind you, palm up, and turn your chin to the **left**. Take the side of your head toward the floor. Some of you will easily touch your head to the floor, while others won't get close. Don't worry about putting your head on the floor. The important aspect of this exercise is folding forward and not touching the floor with your head or sitting on your heels. So don't sit down, fold forward, and stop when your body stops. You have already accomplished the purpose, which is moving your arm and chin in opposite directions and stretching your lower back. If it is extremely awkward kneeling and bending forward, then sit in a chair (without arms) and follow the same instructions.

To come up, press the tops of your feet into the floor to maintain your balance. Start your inhale, lift your sternum (to come up with a flat back), and sweep your **left** arm out to the side and then over your head as you come upright.

Start your exhale by pulling in slightly with your lower abdominal muscles. As you fold forward, sweep your **left** arm behind you while turning your chin toward your **right** shoulder. Inhale, lift your chest, sweep your **right** arm out to the side (pushing your fingertips away from you), and return to kneeling.

Do each side three or four times. Please don't push it too far when you first start practicing. All of these sequences require a slow build up. In the beginning, less is more and more can cause more problems (in other words, pain) than it solves. If you have ever rehabilitated after an injury or surgery, you already know that too much too soon may halt any progress and require you to start all over again.

The next movement requires that you get on your hands and knees. In sanskrit, it is called *cakravakasana* (*cakravaka* = ruddy goose).

CAKRAVAKASANA

TENSION HEADACHE FIG. # 3

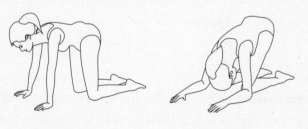

Inhale   *Exhale*

A little padding under your knees may be helpful for this posture. As you inhale, lift your chest without swaying in your lower back. Start your exhale with a slight pulling in of the lower abdom-

inal muscles. Notice that the pulling in of the lower abdominals
lengthens your lower back. Move your buttocks toward your heels
and start folding your chest toward your thighs. Bending your elbows will help you fold forward. If it is easy, take your forehead to
the floor. The exercise is to stretch your lower back, which you have
been compressing in the previous sequence by lifting your chest.
The lower back stretch happens when you fold forward. If you sit
down on your heels before you finish folding forward, you have
missed the lower back stretch. You may have to practice this a few
times to feel the lower back stretch. Repeat *cakravakasana* four or five
times.

BHUJANGASANA (BHUJANGA = COBRA) IS ANOTHER EXERCISE TO STRENGTHEN LOWER BACK MUSCLES

* **Keep in Mind:** Relax your buttocks (gluteus muscles). Lift your
chest, not your chin. When sweeping your arm, push your fingers away
to straighten the arm and open the shoulder.

* **Cautions:** If your shoulders are very tight and sweeping the arms in
bhujangasana causes you more discomfort than relief, omit it. After you
have worked with your shoulders in other asanas for a while, try it
again. Keep your neck long while twisting.

* **Other Benefits:** Greater mobility and range of motion in the neck,
shoulders, and upper and middle back. Strengthens lower back muscles.

Next, lie on the floor on your stomach (prone) for *bhujangasana*
with variations. Place your hands, palms up, in your lower back. If
this isn't comfortable, put your arms at your side, palms up. Put your
right cheek on the floor (your chin is turned toward your left shoul-

der.) As you inhale, lift your chest off the floor, gently but firmly, as high as you comfortably can.

Inhale

It doesn't matter if your chest lifts one inch or six inches off the floor. For now, this is the range of back bending motion in your thoracic (middle and upper) spine. Repetition will increase the flexibility and suppleness in your spine. Any chiropractor will tell you that you are as young as your spine is supple. As you lift your chest, turn your chin to look down at the floor. You are going to do several twists of the neck, so when you lift your chest, **don't** lift your chin. This may take some practice. It seems to be human nature to lift the chest by lifting the chin first. Avoid lifting your chin so that your neck twists comfortably. Lifting your chin scrunches up the back of your neck (cervical vertebra), and it is not healthy or productive to twist your neck while the cervical vertebras are compressed.

Start your exhale; turn your chin toward the left shoulder as you lower your chest back to the floor. Repeat, and lift your chest by inhaling and turn your chin toward the floor. Exhale, lowering your chest while turning your chin in the opposite direction.

Next, start your inhale, then lift your chest and at the same time sweep your **right** arm out to the side, pushing your fingers away, and bring the arm forward. Bend your elbow and touch your forehead with your fingers. It's like a salute. Your face is turned down, looking at the floor.

TENSION HEADACHE FIG. # 5

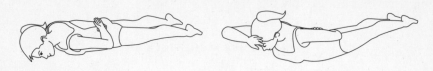

Inhale

Start the exhale; replace your arm behind you as you lower your chest to the floor while turning your chin toward your left shoulder. This sounds complicated, but you will catch on fast. Remember to first start your breath, either an inhale or an exhale, and then begin all of the movements together. To do the other side, start inhaling, then half a second later start all of the movements at the same time—lifting your chest, sweeping your left arm, and turning your chin down. In the beginning, I have found it to be useful, sometimes necessary, to talk myself through asanas such as this. I tell myself to inhale and then tell myself to start all three movements (chest, arm, and chin) all at once.

Do each side three or four times. Remember to start slow. One time on each side may be a good beginning for your body.

*   *   *

Come on to your hands and knees in *cakravakasana*. Exhale, and move your buttocks toward your heels as you fold forward. Repeat four or five times. Until this movement becomes familiar, please see page 29 for instructions.

*   *   *

Now sit and breathe. You can sit in a chair or sit cross-legged on the floor with or without a cushion under your buttocks, whichever is more comfortable for you. The finishing breathing exercise for this sequence is called *sitali*, which is inhaling across your curled, wet tongue and exhaling through your nose. *Sitali* is the only exception to the rule of always inhaling and exhaling through the nose only. In *sitali*, you will inhale across your wet tongue to cool your head and reduce the symptoms of headache.

PRANAYAMA—SITALI

According to the ancient teachers from all traditions, your breath is the key to a healthy, vital life. If you spend even a very short amount of time daily practicing *pranayama* (breath control), it is worth more to you in everyday benefits than all of the vitamins you can swallow.

Simple *pranayama* techniques like *sitali* (use of the tongue to cool the breath) give you the means to balance your entire system.

Curl your tongue by turning the outside edges upward to form a trough, stick your tongue out slightly, and close your lips around the trough. Inhale across your wet tongue, like you are sucking through a straw, gently lifting your chin as you do. At the end of your inhale, curl the tip of your tongue up to touch the soft roof of your mouth, close your lips, and exhale through your nose while gently dropping your chin. Repeat a few times. Feel each breath as it comes and goes.

Use the Basic Breathing Cycle (see page 2)—fill yourself from the top to the bottom, and empty your lungs by gently contracting your lower abdominal muscles below your navel.

Notice the cooling effect of the evaporation of the moisture on your tongue as it calms your system. The gentle lifting and lowering of the chin relaxes the head and neck.

A few people are unable to curl their tongue into a trough. Those people will receive the same cooling effect by slightly opening their lips and teeth, placing the tip of their tongue at the back of their lower teeth, and inhaling across their wet tongue as they follow the other directions for *sitali*.

Finish the sequence by palming your eyes. Close your eyes and place the palms of your hands over your closed eyes for a minute or two. Also, try a little self-examination. Contemplate what gives you the headache in the first place. Your head position while using the computer or the telephone? Your relationship with a coworker or family member? If you can make small adjustments to your physical and emotional environment, you may be able to see big changes in how your body feels and reduce the frequency of tension headaches.

YOUR COMPLETE TENSION HEADACHE SEQUENCE

* * *

Breathing Guidelines

Inhale and exhale through your nose. ∗ Remember to practice ujjayi breathing (control of the breath in the throat). ∗ **On inhale, fill from the top to the bottom.** ∗ As you exhale, empty from the bottom to the top by gently pulling in below the navel. ∗ **Coordinate breathing and moving. Your breath is longer than the movement.** ∗ It starts before the movement and finishes after the movement is completed. ∗

Start ●------------------- B R E A T H -------------------➤ Finish

Start ●-----------M O V E M E N T ----------➤ Finish

See page 4 for details.

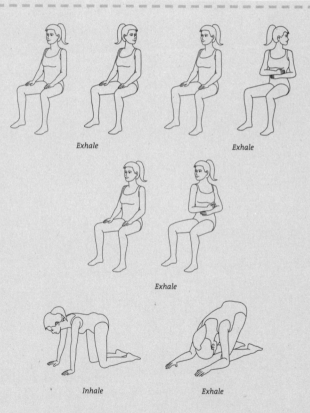

Exhale   Exhale

Exhale

Inhale   Exhale

continued

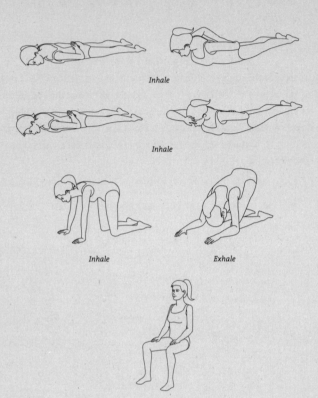

Inhale

Inhale

Inhale   Exhale

Hands and Wrists

You don't have to leave your desk chair to use this sequence, which helps to prevent repetitive motion injuries and carpal tunnel disorder. Gentle movement and stretching greatly increases blood flow and the movement of life force energy while relieving stiffness and the negative effects of repetitive motion. Moving your fingers and wrists in their full range of motion will help eliminate soreness and reduce the effects of natural aging in your hands.

Steve, a friend of mine, is a professional drummer who tours regularly with a well-known rock band. One day he told me that his hands and wrists were starting to stiffen up. After his nearly twenty years of playing drums for a living, I was not surprised. The same exercises that brought him great relief are in this chapter. Other students, including a computer programmer and a graphic artist, have also used them with success.

HANDS AND WRISTS IN MOTION

* **Keep in Mind:** Open on inhale. Close on exhale.

* **Cautions:** Don't use too much force. Open and close firmly but gently. Don't overdo this exercise. A few times each session two or three times a day is plenty to start.

* **Other Benefits:** Increased manual dexterity.

Sit up straight in your chair, hands in your lap, and breathe. You can have your eyes open or closed. First, feel your breath come and go a few times. Then take your attention and your breath to your hands. With each inhale, imagine sending your breath down your arms to the tips of your fingers.

HANDS AND WRISTS EXERCISE FIG. # 1

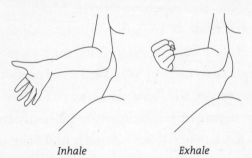

Inhale   Exhale

- Feel your fingers and hands.

- Relax your shoulders, arms, wrists, and hands.

- Now, slowly, as you inhale, open your hands, and spread your fingers as wide as they will go.

- Exhale and very gently but firmly, starting with the little fingers, close your fingers into a fist.

- Next, inhale, and starting with your thumbs, open one finger at a time, then bend your wrists back as far as they will comfortably go.

- With your next exhale, close the fists, starting with the little fingers, and fold your fists forward to stretch your wrists in the opposite direction.

- Repeat three or four times, open your fists on the inhale and bend your wrists back, and then close the fists on exhale while folding your wrists forward.

- Sit, breathe, and feel your fingers, hands, and wrists. They feel more alive, don't they? In addition, there should be a feeling of openness and suppleness.

The next step is to move these stress relieving benefits throughout your shoulders, upper back, and neck. While working the hands, you will add sweeping your arms up over your head and then bring the hands down alternately to the chest, and then behind the back. The arm motion moves the effect from the fingers through the arms to the upper back and neck. Just a few times during the day brings great relief.

HAND AND WRISTS AND SHOULDER EXERCISE

* **Keep in Mind:** Start your breath, and then start sweeping your arms. Push your hands away from you to straighten and lengthen your arms and open your shoulders.

* **Cautions:** Start slow. Three or four repetitions, two or three times a day is enough to start.

* **Other Benefits:** A great "time out" from any task. Clears your head to promote better problem solving.

• Sit, breathe, and feel your fingers and hands.

• Relax your shoulders, arms, wrists, and hands.

• Now, as you inhale, slowly open your hands and spread your fingers as wide as they will go, then bend your wrists back *while sweeping your arms out to the side and up over your head*. (Begin your inhale and then start all of the movements simultaneously, arms sweeping, fingers, hands, and wrists opening.)

• Exhale, close your fingers into a fist, starting with the little fingers, and fold your wrist forward, while bringing your arms down and your hands together at your chest.

• Next, begin your inhale, then start sweeping your arms and opening your hands and bending the wrists backward. Take your arms up over your head.

• Exhale, lower your arms, and take your hands *behind your back* as you close your fists and fold your wrists forward.

This is a similar arm movement to the one you used in the Your Neck exercise (page 13).

YOUR COMPLETE HANDS AND WRISTS AND SHOULDERS SEQUENCE

* * *

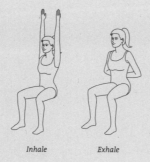

Inhale   Exhale

Repeat three or four times, alternating bringing your hands in front and behind you.

Sit, breathe and feel your hands, arms, shoulders, and upper back. They feel more alive, don't they? Also, there will be a feeling of openness and suppleness in your shoulders, back, and neck.

Knees

Two friends, both former professional athletes, complained of constant pain in their left knees. Coincidentally, they both drove SUVs with standard transmissions. Constantly working the clutch severely aggravated their less-than-healthy knees. Out of familiarity, the shifting went unsuspected as a possible cause of their discomfort. I knew what the problem was. First, I told them to buy a new car. Once they had automatic transmissions, they eliminated a lot of wear and tear on their knees. Then we began a rehabilitation sequence to strengthen the connective tissue above and below the knee without straining or twisting the joint itself.

APANASANA AND SUPTA EKA PADANGUSTHASANA

* **Keep in Mind:** Move with your breath. Flex the feet as you raise the legs. Keep your chin down.

* **Cautions:** People with a Lumbar Disk That Is Currently "Bulging" Should Not Straighten Their Legs in This Position.

* **Other Benefits:** Helps stretch hamstring muscles and calf. Increases ankle mobility.

The first posture is *apanasana* (*apana* = vital air of the lower abdomen). Use your yoga mat and lie on your back with knees bent and feet lifted. Place your hands *on the backs of your legs, just below the knees.* Exhale, and gently pull the thighs toward the chest. Inhale, and straighten your arms by pushing your thighs away. Repeat a few times to warm up the lower back.

KNEES FIG. # 1

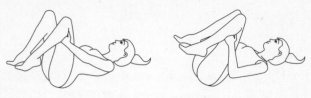

Exhale

As you exhale, pull in. On inhale, push away. Coordinate the movement with your breathing. Remember the short pauses that happen at the end of the exhale and the end of the inhale. Begin your exhale and then start pulling your legs in. Finish the movement, finish the breath, and feel the short (half-second) pause. Then start your inhale, straighten your arms, and come to a full stop. Repeat four or five times.

If it seems like a long distance from the back of your head to the floor, a small pillow or a folded towel will make this position more comfortable and productive. Focus your attention to your lower back and think of breathing into it. Attention plus breath equals awareness. Awareness of what is happening in your body is half the battle. Awareness will ease your path to a supple, strong body and greatly reduce the risk of injury.

SUPTA EKA PADANGUSTHASANA

For *supta* (as in supine) *eka* (one) *padangusthasana* (*padagustha* = big toe, *padagusthasana* = hold toe posture), but we will forego the fingers on the big toe and just straighten the leg.

Keep your hands behind your legs, inhale, and straighten one leg toward the ceiling. Then exhale and bend the knee. **Alternate** legs to stretch the hamstrings, calves, and Achilles tendon.

KNEES FIG. # 2

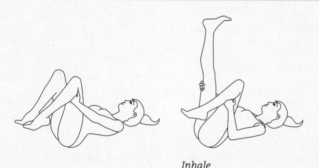

Inhale

Work with your breath, not against it. Straighten your leg on inhale and bend your knee on exhale. Repeat three or four times with each leg.

Then, straighten both legs at the same time. Repeat three or four times.

* * *

DVIPADA PITHAM

* **Keep in Mind:** Keep your head down, chin toward the chest. Move with your breath.

* **Cautions:** Keep your lower back long, not compressed.

* **Other Benefits:** Mobility in middle back. Traction effect for the neck.

The next asana is *dvipada pitham* (*dvipada* = two feet, *pitham* = pose). Lie on your back with your arms at your sides. Bend your knees with your feet flat on the floor. With your thighs comfortably apart, place your heels under your knees.

KNEES FIG. # 3

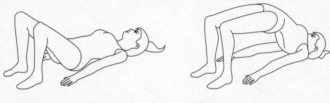

Inhale

• Lengthen or flatten your lower back against the floor.

• As you inhale, push down with your feet and push your hips up, lifting your spine off the floor vertebra by vertebra. Keep your chin down to lengthen your neck. Come to a full stop.

• Exhale and roll down, vertebra by vertebra. It is as if your spine is a string of pearls and you are lifting and then putting them down, one pearl at a time.

• Keep your lower back long so that your lumbar spine touches the floor before your buttocks.

• Repeat four to six times. Use *ujjayi* breathing (page 5) and listen for the sound of your breath in your throat. Your breath will tell you how your body is reacting to this backward bending pose.

Repeat *apanasana* four or five times with your hands behind your knees as before.

KNEES FIG. # 4

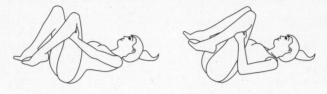

Exhale

---

*   *   *

ARDHA SALABHASANA

*   **Keep in Mind:** Lift the leg only three or four inches off the floor. It's not necessary to lift any higher.

*   **Cautions:** If holding the leg off the floor while bending the knee causes stress in the lower back, omit this asana. To strengthen lower back muscles, see the chapter on lower back. *Do not* push down with your hands or arms. Lift the chest with back muscles, not arm muscles.

*   **Other Benefits:** Strengthens lower back.

The next posture is *ardha salabhasana* (*ardha* = half, *salabhasana* = locust). While lying on the stomach, lift one leg, bend the knee, then straighten the leg and lower it back to the floor.

KNEES FIG. # 5

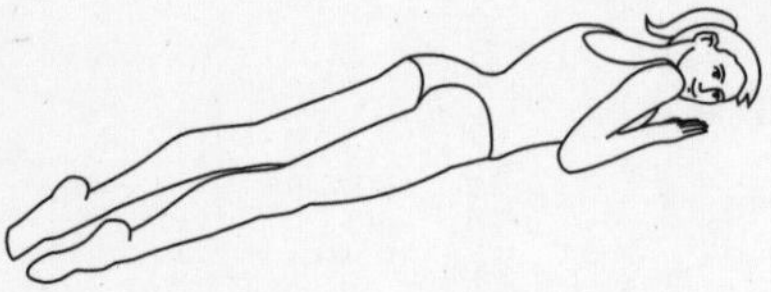

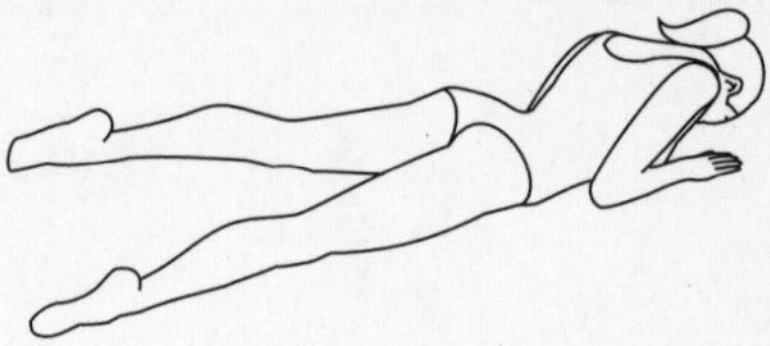

Inhale

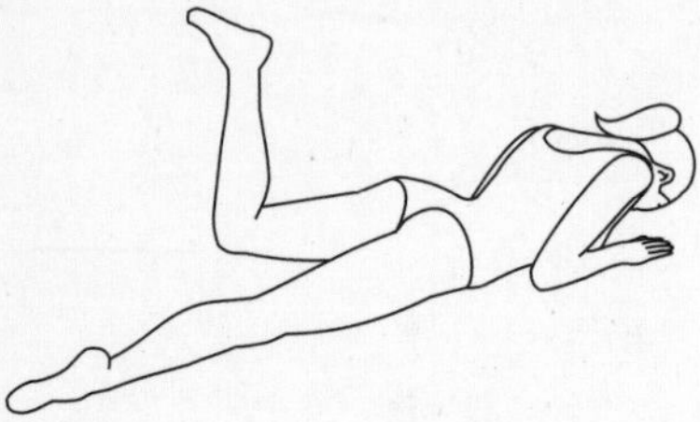

Exhale

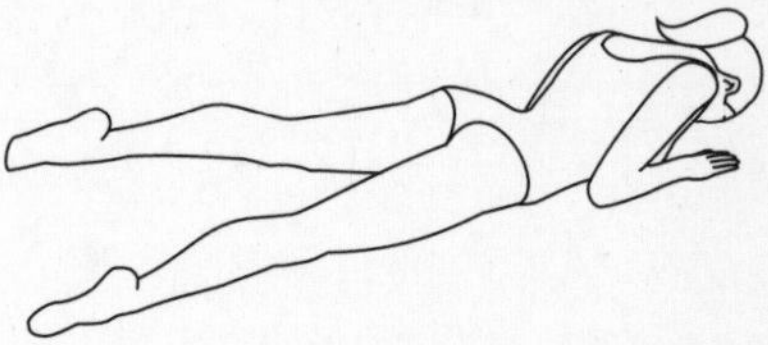

Inhale

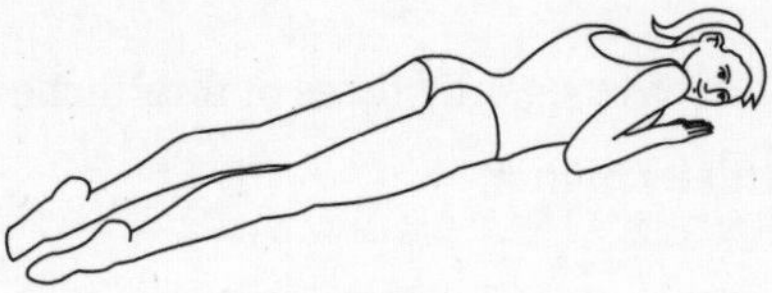

Exhale

While lying on your stomach (prone) with your elbows bent, hands or forearms on the floor, *turn your chin toward your **right** shoulder, placing your **left** cheek on the floor.* As you inhale, lift your chest and straight left leg while turning your face to the floor. Keep your leg up, exhale, and bend your left knee. Inhale, then straighten the left leg. Exhale; lower your leg and chest. Turn your chin to the left. Repeat with your right leg. Alternate sides three or four times to start.

*   *   *

Repeat *apanasana* four or five times with your hands behind your knees as before.

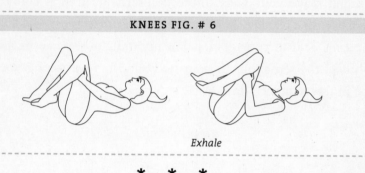

Exhale

* * *

SUPTA EKA PADANGUSTHASANA

Lie on your back with your hands behind your knees, inhale, and straighten both legs, pushing your heels toward the ceiling. Exhale and bend your legs. Repeat four or five times.

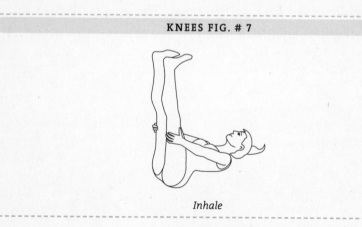

Inhale

* * *

SAVASANA

When you finish, lie on your back on your yoga mat for a few minutes in *savasana* (*sava* = corpse posture). This is where it all comes together. Get comfortable. Use a small pillow or towel under your head. A pillow or bolster under your knees will lengthen your lower back and make your knees more comfortable. If it is chilly, cover yourself with a blanket. Allow three to five minutes if possible. Bring your arms next to your sides, palms up, and close your eyes. Breathe easily, feel the sensations in your body, and let everything you have done in this sequence sink in.

KNEES FIG. # 8

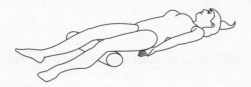

These postures strengthen the musculature of the legs around the knee, especially at the back of the knees. The goal is *sthira*—stability—in this case for knees that have paid the price of hard use.

YOUR COMPLETE KNEES SEQUENCE

* * *

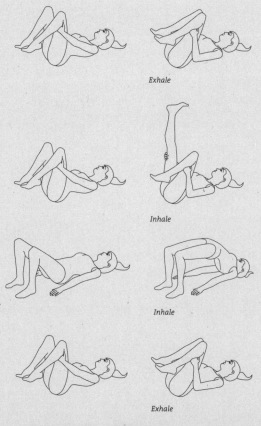

Exhale

Inhale

Inhale

Exhale

continued

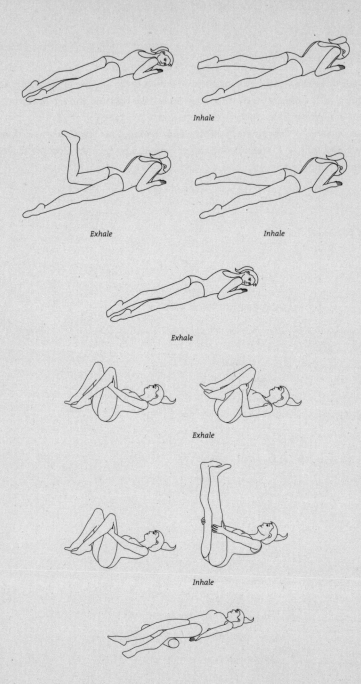

Inhale

Exhale   Inhale

Exhale

Exhale

Inhale

6

Upper Back and Shoulders

Do you hunch over your desk five days a week? Are you on the computer all day? Do you drive a vehicle leaning forward to the steering wheel, or bend over, as a nurse or dental hygienist does, in service to patients? If your work requires you to deepen the curve of the thoracic (upper and middle) spine and you don't want to look like a camel before you're fifty-five, back bends are called for. Regardless of your age or physical condition, a helpful and preventative series of easy back-bending postures to open your chest and help avoid a deeply rounded and painful back can be done lying down, sitting, and standing up.

To begin, get some movement in this area by doing the second sequence in the Your Neck chapter (page 13) but, instead of sitting, do the movements standing up. Stand on your yoga mat, with your arms at your side and your feet about hip-width apart. Be balanced on your feet. Feel yourself to be stable. Close your eyes and breathe. Also, remember to use *ujjayi* breathing (see page 5), which is the control of the breath in the throat. Feel your chest rise with your inhale and slightly drop with your exhale. Picture your back in your mind's eye. Begin to feel your back move as you breathe. As you slightly deepen your inhale, feel your chest lift and the roundness in your back flatten just a bit. Take a few more breaths with your awareness on how your back feels.

Open your eyes and bring your palms together at your chest with your elbows pointing down toward the floor. Inhale, open your arms, exhale, and close your arms. Repeat three or four times. Next, inhale, open your arms, and keep them open as you exhale. Inhale, gently lift your chest, and pull your shoulders back a little farther. Do not compress or collapse in the lower back. Keep it lengthened. Take two or three more breaths and then release. Go back to the start position and lower your arms. Stand, breathe, and feel your back.

YOUR BACK

UPPER BACK FIG. # 1

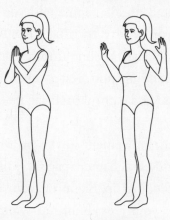

Inhale

YOUR BACK AND SHOULDERS

* **Keep in Mind:** When sweeping your arms, push your fingertips away to straighten the arms and open the shoulders. Start your exhale by gently pulling in below your navel.

* **Cautions:** Do not force your arms to move farther than your shoulders will allow at first.

* **Other Benefits:** Increased mobility in shoulders.

Return to the start position, palms together at your chest. With your next inhale, open and extend your arms as you sweep them out to the side, and then bring them up over your head. Come to a full stop. Exhale and lower your arms—take your hands behind you and turn your palms so that the backs of your hands rest in the lower back area. Feel your arm bones (humerus) rotate in your shoulder as you lower your arms. Repeat three or four times.

UPPER BACK FIG. # 2

Exhale   Inhale   Exhale   Inhale   Exhale

VIRABHADRASANA

* **Keep in Mind:** At the start position, lengthen your lower back by dropping the tail bone, lifting the pubic bone, and making a slight backward tilt of the pelvis.

* **Cautions:** Do not collapse or compress your lower back.

* **Other Benefits:** Opens the chest and shoulders. Builds leg strength.

Virabhadrasana (*virabhadra* = a hero, *asana* = posture = warrior posture) will help your back. Stand with one foot forward, feet at hips width and interlace your fingers behind your back, elbows slightly bent. As you inhale, bend your front knee and simultaneously straighten and lift your arms behind you. Exhale and return to the start position.

UPPER BACK FIG. # 3

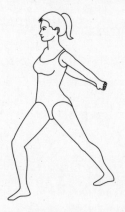

Inhale

Repeat three or four times, then hold the second position for two or three breaths. Repeat with the other foot forward. Then stand with your arms at your side and feel your back.

CAKRAVAKASANA

Come on to your hands and knees into *cakravakasana* (see page 29). Exhale and move your buttocks toward your heels as you fold forward. Repeat four or five times.

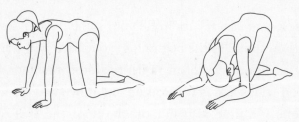

UPPER BACK FIG. # 4

Exhale

*   *   *

DVIPADA PITHAM

* **Keep in Mind:** When you roll up, lengthen your neck by dropping your head and chin toward your sternum.

* **Cautions:** Keep your lower back long, not compressed.

* **Other Benefits:** Flexibility and suppleness in the spine.

The next asana is *dvipada pitham* (two feet pose; see page 45.) This time, the pose is utilized to bend your back backward.

• Lie on your back with your arms at your sides. Bend your knees with your feet flat on the floor. With your thighs comfortably apart, place your heels under your knees.

• Lengthen or flatten your lower back against the floor.

• As you inhale, push down with your feet and push your hips up, lifting your spine off the floor vertebra by vertebra. Keep your chin down to lengthen your neck. Come to a full stop with the movement and your breath.

• Exhale and roll down, vertebra by vertebra. Keep your lower back long so that your lumbar spine touches the floor before your buttocks.

As best as you can, try to "roll" your spine up and down. Try to articulate your spine. In the beginning, your back will want to move all at once, as if you were lifting a flat board off the floor. Keep your attention on your back as you roll up and down and try to feel each vertebra, one at a time, as it lifts off the floor and as it touches the floor on the way down. Repeat four to six times.

UPPER BACK FIG. # 5

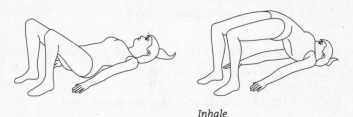

Inhale

*   *   *

APANASANA AND SUPTA EKA
PADANGUSTHASANA VARIATION

Here, *apanasana* is used as a counterpose to stretch your lower back. Coordinate the movement with your breathing. Use the short pauses that happen at the end of the exhale and the end of the inhale to come to a full stop. That means to begin your exhale and then start pulling in. Finish the movement, finish the breath, and feel the short (half-second) pause. Then, start your inhale, straighten your arms, and come to a full stop. Repeat four or five times, then hug your thighs to your chest for a few breaths. Remember to use a small pillow or a folded towel under your head if it makes you more comfortable.

- Lie on your back with your knees bent and feet lifted.

- Place one hand on **each kneecap**. As you exhale, pull your thighs toward your chest. Keep your hands on your kneecaps.

- As you inhale, push your knees away.

UPPER BACK FIG. # 6

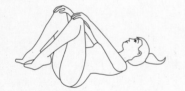 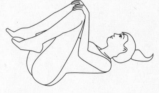

Exhale

*   *   *

*   **Keep in mind:** Move with your breath. Flex your feet as you raise your legs. Keep your chin down.

*   **Cautions:** People with a Lumbar Disk That Is Currently "Bulging" Should Not Straighten Their Legs in This Position. Don't force your arms to the floor; be easy on your shoulders.

*   **Other Benefits:** Helps to stretch hamstring and calf muscles. Increases ankle mobility.

From the apanasana position, inhale, straighten your legs, push your heels toward the ceiling, and lift your arms up over your head. Try to bring your fingertips to the floor behind you. Exhale, bend your knees, lower your arms, and hug your knees. Repeat two or three times, then hug your knees for a couple of breaths.

UPPER BACK FIG. # 7

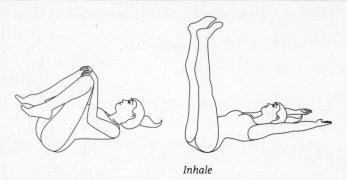

Inhale

* * *

SAVASANA

When you finish, lie back on your yoga mat for a few minutes of *savasana* (corpse posture). Get comfortable. You can use a small pillow or towel under your head. If it is chilly, cover yourself with a blanket. Allow three to five minutes, if possible. Bring your arms next to your sides with your palms up, and close your eyes. Breathe easily and feel the sensations in your body. Let all of the work you have done sink in.

YOUR BACK FIG. # 8

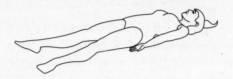

After *savasana*, if you have a few minutes to spare, sit up straight in a chair or on your mat and breathe. Visualize your spine. As you inhale, feel your sternum gently lift and "see" your thoracic spine slightly flatten out. "See" how your inhale lengthens and straightens your back. As you exhale, "see" and feel the curve deepen again. Use this visualization to create more articulation in your spine.

YOUR COMPLETE UPPER BACK
AND SHOULDERS SEQUENCE

* * *

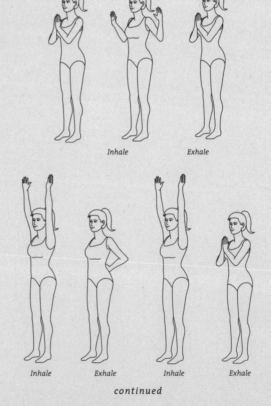

Inhale   Exhale

Inhale   Exhale   Inhale   Exhale

continued

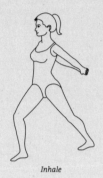

Inhale

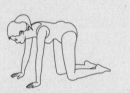

Inhale

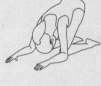

Exhale

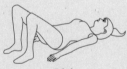

Exhale

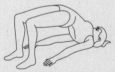

Inhale

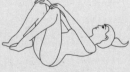

Inhale

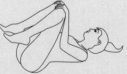

Exhale

continued

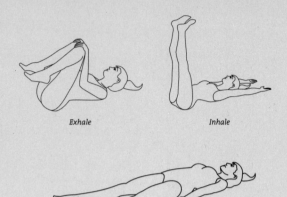

Exhale   *Inhale*

7

Lower Back—Lumbar Spine

One of my students is an elementary school teacher. When she teaches fifth and sixth graders, her lower back does not bother her. When she teaches second and third graders, her back gives her a lot of grief. Why? The younger students are smaller. So are their desks. She must stoop over to assist the shorter kids. When she began coming to my class, I knew what grade she had been teaching that week by the condition of her back. During our work together, she has made significant progress in strengthening her lower back.

What is the cure for lower back discomfort? The party line in the gym is that strong abdominal muscles will take care of your lower back. That is only half of the truth. Without specific exercise, the average person has both tight and weak muscles in his or her lower back. Just as you would strengthen your biceps by lifting a dumbbell (contracting the muscle and then lowering the dumbbell, stretching the muscle), the same technique of contracting and stretching creates a supple, strong lower back. After a few gentle forward bends, such as hugging your knees to your chest to prepare the muscles, a sequence of stronger asanas are called for. Back bends that contract, and forward bends that stretch, are used in conjunction with the weight of the torso itself to bring health and vitality to the lower back. The position of the arms is used to add or subtract weight, as you would add additional weight to the dumbbell, to progressively increase your strength, flexibility, and, most important, stability in the lumbar area.

Front leg lifts, done on the floor, are added to strengthen the core torso muscles in the abdomen. In the chapter on the lower back and sacrum, backward leg lifts are added to further strengthen the muscles in the lumbar/sacrum area.

APANASANA

* **Keep in Mind:** Keep your shoulders on the floor. Keep your hands on the kneecaps. Coordinate breath and movement.

* **Cautions:** Do not pull too hard; this is a warm-up.

* **Other Benefits:** Will increase range of motion in hips.

• Lie on your back on your yoga mat.

• Bend your knees and lift your feet. Place one hand on **each kneecap**.

• As you exhale, gently but firmly pull your thighs toward your chest. Keep your hands on your kneecaps.

• As you inhale, push your knees away.

• Coordinate the movement with your breathing. Remember the short pauses that happen at the end of the exhale and the end of the inhale. That means start your exhale and then start pulling in. Finish the movement, finish the breath, and feel the short (half-second) pause.

- Use *ujjayi* breathing (see page 5). Control your breath in your throat and listen to the sound of your breathing. Then, start your inhale, straighten your arms, and come to a full stop.

LOWER BACK—LUMBAR FIG. # 1

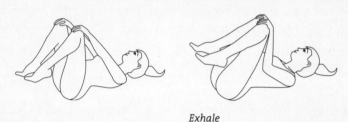

Exhale

Repeat four or five times. Use a small pillow or a folded towel under your head to make this position more comfortable and productive. Focus your attention to your lower back and think of breathing into it. Attention plus breath equals awareness. Awareness of what is happening in your body is half the battle. Awareness will ease your path to a supple, strong body and greatly reduce the risk of injury.

*   *   *

SUPTA EKA PADANGUSTHASANA

Supta (as in supine), *eka* (one), *Padangusthasana* (padagustha = big toe; and padagusthasana = hold toe posture). We will forego the fingers on the big toe and just straighten the leg.

- **Keep in Mind:** Flex the foot as you raise the leg. Keep your chin down.

- **Cautions:** People with a Lumbar Disk That Is Currently "Bulging" Should Not Straighten Their Legs in This Position.

- **Other Benefits:** Helps to stretch hamstring and calf muscles. Increases ankle mobility.

• Place one hand behind each leg just below your knee.

• Inhale and straighten your **right** leg. Push the heel up toward the ceiling and pull your toes back to flex your ankle. Come to a full stop, both moving and breathing.

• Start your exhale, then start bending your knee and pointing your toes. Come to a full stop.

• Inhale, straighten your **left** leg.

Repeat four or five times with each leg. Use a small pillow or folded towel behind your head if that is more comfortable for you.

LOWER BACK—LUMBAR FIG. # 2

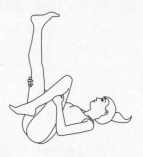

Inhale

* * *

CAKRAVAKASANA

Come onto your hands and knees for *cakravakasana* (see page 29). Exhale and move your buttocks toward your heels as you fold forward. Repeat four or five times.

LOWER BACK—LUMBAR FIG. # 3

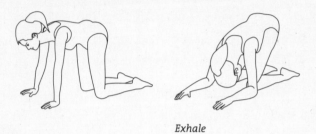

Exhale

* * *

BHUJANGASANA

* **Keep in Mind:** Lift your chest, not your chin, on inhale.

* **Cautions:** Do not tense up your gluteus (buttocks).

* **Other Benefits:** Opens front of the chest. Increases neck mobility.

Each successive pose provides more work for the muscles of the lower back. The first lifts the chest off the floor, which bends the thoracic spine backward and contracts, thus strengthening the lumbar area muscles. The second pose adds sweeping one arm and bending the elbow while lifting the chest off the floor, which adds the weight of the arm to the load the back muscles must carry. The third uses a straight arm to increase the length and weight of what is being lifted off the floor. Adding arms to the movement is how you gradually increase the weight of your torso to strengthen the muscles in the lower back.

Lie on your yoga mat, face down, one cheek on the floor, with your palms turned up in your lower back. Inhale, lift your chest, not your chin, and gently but firmly come up as high as you can. Exhale and lower your chest while turning your chin in the opposite direction.

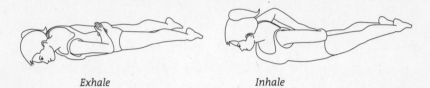

Exhale   *Inhale*

It does not matter how high your chest comes off the floor. Repetition will increase the flexibility in your spine. Start now to increase your spine's suppleness while strengthening the muscles in your lower back. Repeat four times.

CAKRAVAKASANA

To stretch and relieve your lower back, push yourself up to hands and knees and repeat cakravakasana (see page 29) three times.

BHUJANGASANA WITH A SALUTE

* **Keep in Mind:** Keep your buttocks (gluteus muscles) relaxed. Lift your chest, not your chin. When sweeping your arm, push your fingers away to straighten the arm and open the shoulder.

* **Cautions:** If your shoulders are very tight and sweeping the arms in bhujangasana causes you more discomfort than relief, omit it. After you have worked with your shoulders in other asanas for a while, try it again. Keep your neck long while twisting.

* **Other Benefits:** Greater mobility and range of motion in the neck, shoulders, and upper and middle back. Strengthens lower back muscles.

Lie on your yoga mat, face down, *left* cheek on the floor, with palms turned up in your lower back. Inhale, lift your chest, not your chin, and sweep your *right* arm forward, bending the elbow and touching your fingers to your forehead. Gently but firmly come up as high as you can. Exhale; lower your chest, replace your arm behind you while turning your chin in the opposite direction. Repeat with the opposite arm. Do each side two or three times.

LOWER BACK—LUMBAR FIG. # 5

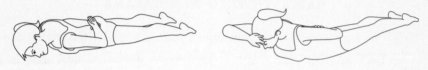

Inhale

Repeat *cakravakasana* (see page 29) three times.

BHUJANGASANA WITH SWEEPING ARMS

* **Keep in Mind:** Keep your buttocks (gluteus muscles) relaxed. Lift your chest, not your chin. When sweeping your arm, push your fingers away to straighten the arm and open the shoulder.

* **Cautions:** If after one repetition it feels as if your lower back is doing too much too soon, bend your elbow until you have built more strength in your lower back.

* **Other Benefits:** Greater mobility and range of motion in the neck, shoulders, and upper and middle back.

Next, lie on your stomach again and repeat *bhujangasana* while sweeping your **straight** arm forward and up to your ear. It takes much stronger lower back muscles to lift the chest and sweep a straight arm forward than it does to lift only your chest. ***Avoid starting with the most difficult variation.*** It's like going to the gym and trying to bench press 300 pounds the first time. You may be sorry that you tried too much, too fast. Add more weight (arm position) slowly over days as you build up strength.

Repeat *cakravakasana* (see page 29) three times.

SAMASTHITI TO UTTANASANA

This Vinyasa, *samasthiti* to *uttanasana*, stretches and strengthens the lower back muscles. *Samasthiti* (*sama* = equal, *sthiti* = stable, equal stability posture); *uttanasana* (*uttana* = upright, stretched out = upright stretch posture).

The most important bit of information to remember is that *bending your knees* is the **safety valve** for your lower back. Start folding forward then let your knees bend slightly also. Keep your knees slightly bent until you are all the way back up to the standing position. The movement creates much less strain in the lower back muscles with the knees bent. Thus, this repetition is much more beneficial with your knees bent, especially to the beginning practitioner.

Also, let's revisit the idea of arm placement to add or subtract weight to what is being lifted. The illustration instructs you to hold your arms up by your ears as you bend forward and as you lift back up to the standing position. This is the **most challenging position**. You may want to start by bending forward and sliding your hands down the backs of your legs and coming up by lifting your chest and sliding your hands up the backs of your legs. This is the least amount of weight your lower back has to carry.

Next time try sweeping the arms to the side, which adds the

weight of the arms. Holding your arms by your ears adds weight and length to the load. Please start slowly with two or three repetitions and don't use your arms. If that seems very easy on your lower back, tomorrow do two or three more, this time sweeping your arms. Get some experience under your belt of how your lower back reacts before moving on to holding your arms by your ears. After you have built up some strength and flexibility in your lower back, it will be no big deal.

LOWER BACK—LUMBAR FIG. # 6

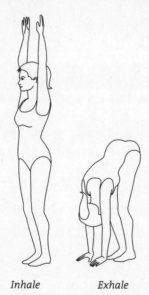

Inhale   *Exhale*

---

* **Keep in Mind:** Start your exhale by pulling in below the navel. To return to the standing position, inhale and lift your chest to come up with a flat back.

* **Cautions:** Avoid lifting your chin on inhale.

* **Other Benefits:** Stretches hamstring muscles.

• Stand on your yoga mat. Have your feet hip-width apart or wide enough to keep your balance as you bend forward and come up.

• Inhale and stand tall. Do not lift your arms the first time you try this posture. Instead, put your hands on your buttocks.

• Exhale, gently pull in below the navel, fold forward (leading with your heart, not your chin), bend your knees slightly, and slide your hands down the back of your legs.

• To return to the standing position, inhale, lift your chest up and away from your thighs, and slide your hands up the back of your legs.

UTTANASANA WITH ARMS

• Stand with feet hip-distance apart. Inhale; sweep your arms out to the side and over your head.

• Exhale; pull in below the navel and fold forward, bending the knees slightly as you sweep your arms down. Bend your knees enough to touch the floor with your fingers.

• Keep the bend in your knees, inhale, and lift your chest as you sweep your arms to the side. Return to the standing position, lifting your arms over your head.

• Exhale and lower your arms to your side.

After you have practiced these first two versions for a while, try it with your arms coming forward rather than out to the side. Always bend your knees. Go slow!

VIRABHADRASANA

* **Keep in Mind:** Stay balanced on your feet. Keep your elbows pointing down toward the floor.

* **Cautions:** Do not bounce on your front knee when you straighten the leg. Avoid compressing the lower back.

* **Other Benefits:** Expands chest and flattens upper back. Increases shoulder mobility. Strengthens your leg muscles.

Virabhadrasana (*virabhadra* = a hero, *asana* = posture, warrior posture). This posture can also be done sitting in a chair (see page 56).

Stand with one foot forward, feet as wide as your hips, and palms together at your chest. Inhale; simultaneously bend the front knee and, keeping your elbows down, open your forearms. Exhale; straighten the front leg as you close your forearms back together. Repeat three times, then switch legs and repeat.

LOWER BACK—LUMBAR FIG. # 7

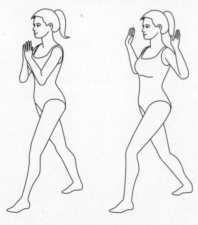

Inhale

Come down to hands and knees to *cakravakasana* (see page 29). Exhale, move your buttocks toward your heels as you fold forward. Inhale, lift your chest, and return to hands and knees. Repeat four or five times.

APANASANA

Lie on your back. Repeat apanasana (see page 44) three or four times. Bend your knees and lift your feet. Place one hand on each kneecap. As you exhale, pull your thighs toward your chest. Keep your hands on your kneecaps and, as you inhale, push your knees away.

SUPTA EKA PADANGUSTHASANA VARIATION

* **Keep in Mind:** Move with your breath—use longer, slower breathing.

* **Cautions:** One repetition may be enough to start. Keep your awareness in your lower back. Don't do too much too soon.

* **Other Benefits:** Increases hip mobility.

LOWER BACK—LUMBAR FIG. # 8

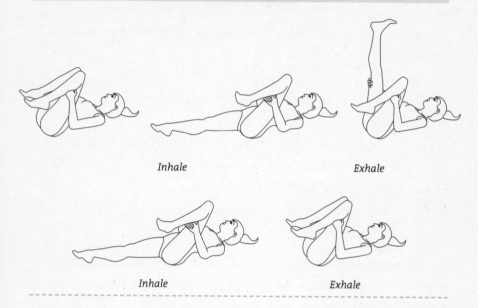

Inhale   *Exhale*

Inhale   *Exhale*

Bend your knees with your feet off the floor and both hands holding your **left** leg. On inhale, straighten your **right** leg, keeping it close to but not on the floor. Exhale; lift the foot toward the ceiling. Inhale; lower the leg down (keep the foot off the floor). Exhale; bend the knee, returning to the starting position. Repeat three or four times, then do the same thing with the other leg. When you finish, hug your knees for a few breaths. This is important to stretch out your lower back.

APANASANA

Repeat *apanasana* three or four times, and then hug your thighs to your chest for a few breaths.

SAVASANA

When you finish, lie back on your yoga mat for a few minutes of *savasana*.

LOWER BACK—LUMBAR FIG. # 9

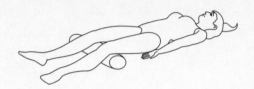

Get comfortable. Use a small pillow or towel under your head. A pillow or bolster under your knees will lengthen your lower back. If it is chilly, cover yourself with a blanket. Allow three to five minutes if possible. Bring your arms next to your sides, palms up, and close your eyes. Breathe easily, feel the sensations in your body, and let everything you have done in this sequence jell.

Avoid the most challenging versions of the asanas when you begin practicing. Even going slowly, using this sequence will quickly bring strength and suppleness to your lower back.

YOUR COMPLETE LOWER BACK— LUMBAR SPINE SEQUENCE.

* * *

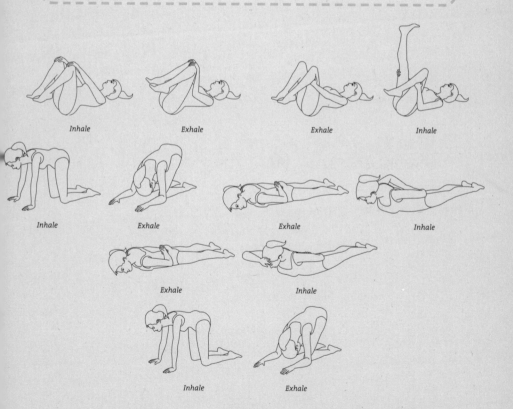

Inhale   Exhale   Exhale   Inhale

Inhale   Exhale   Exhale   Inhale

Exhale   Inhale

Inhale   Exhale

continued

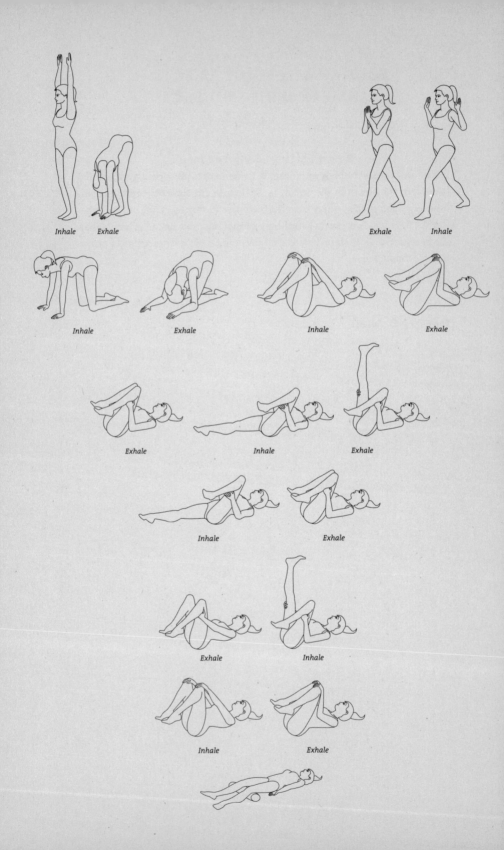

Inhale   Exhale   Exhale   Inhale

Inhale   Exhale   Inhale   Exhale

Exhale   Inhale   Exhale

Inhale   Exhale

Exhale   Inhale

Inhale   Exhale

8

Lower Back—Sacroiliac

A congenital condition, such as having legs of a different length or a tendency toward scoliosis of the spine, can often create physical discomfort. However, habitual musculoskeletal misuse and overuse also leads to painful conditions.

If you have lower back discomfort and you don't know why, try looking at how you use your body. Stand up on both feet and balance your weight. Now slouch to the side where you habitually slouch. Next, slouch on the other side. This will feel weird because you never slouch on that side—you favor one side over the other just as a woman usually carries her purse on the same shoulder, her young child on the same hip, and a man puts his wallet in the same back pocket and sits on it all day, year after year. Human beings are creatures of habit. When we use yoga to change our habits and to balance the way we use our bodies, many painful conditions are greatly improved.

I have had challenges with my lower back for more than thirty-five years. In my right sacroiliac joint, I have shear stress where the sacrum and ilium meet. Following are the asanas prescribed to me by my yoga teacher twelve years ago. I have used them almost daily to relieve lower back pain. Nearly daily maintenance is the key.

When I keep my lower back muscles strong and supple, I have no problems.

This chapter addresses the sacroiliac joint, the junction of the ilium (hipbone) and the sacrum (the triangular shaped wedge of five-fused vertebra at the base of the spine between the two hipbones).

APANASANA

* **Keep in Mind:** Keep your shoulders on the floor. Keep your hands on your kneecaps. Coordinate breath and movement.

* **Cautions:** Do not pull too hard, as this is a warm-up.

* **Other Benefits:** Will increase range of motion in hips.

Strength and stability are our goal. Let's begin on the floor for apanasana. Lie on your back on your yoga mat. Bend your knees and lift your feet. Place one hand on each kneecap. As you exhale, gently but firmly pull your thighs toward your chest. Keep your hands on your kneecaps as you inhale, then push your knees away.

LOWER BACK—SACROILIAC FIG. #1

Inhale   Exhale

Coordinate the movement with your breathing. Remember the short pauses that happen at the end of the exhale and the end of the inhale. That means start your exhale and then start pulling in. Finish the movement, finish the breath, and feel the short (half second) pause. Then, start your inhale, straighten your arms, and come to a full stop. Repeat four or five times. Use *ujjayi* (see page 5) breathing to control your breath in your throat. A small pillow or a folded towel behind your head will make this position more comfortable and productive. Focus your attention on your lower back and breathe into it. Attention plus breath equals awareness. Awareness of what is happening in your body is half the battle. Awareness will ease your path to a supple, strong body and greatly reduce the risk of injury.

SUPTA EKA PADANGUSTHASANA

* **Keep in Mind:** Flex the foot as you raise the leg. Keep your chin down.

* **Cautions:** People with a Lumbar Disk That Is Currently "Bulging" Should Not Straighten Their Legs in This Position.

* **Other Benefits:** Helps to stretch hamstring and calf muscles. Increases ankle mobility.

Next, place one hand behind each leg just below your knee. Inhale and straighten **one** leg. Push the heel up toward the ceiling and pull your toes back to flex your ankle. Come to a full stop. Start your exhale, then start bending your knee and pointing your toes. Come to a full stop. Inhale, straighten your **other** leg. Repeat four or five times with each leg.

LOWER BACK—SACROILIAC FIG. #2

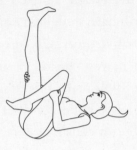

Inhale

Come on to your hands and knees into *cakravakasana* (see page 29). Exhale, then move your buttocks toward your heels as you fold forward. Repeat four or five times.

LOWER BACK—SACROILIAC FIG. # 3

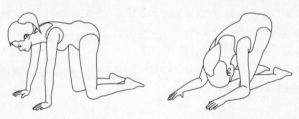

Inhale   *Exhale*

Learning Tool—Hip Rotation

Sit on your yoga mat with your knees bent and your feet on the floor. Lean back onto your elbows. Lift one leg, straighten it, and turn your toes inward; then turn your toes outward. Notice that this rotation is happening at the top of the leg (femur) bone in your hip joint, not at your knee or ankle. This is inward or outward hip rotation.

VIMANASANA

* **Keep in Mind:** Use an *inward rotation* of your hips. As you inhale, lift one leg, and as you exhale, lower the leg to the floor.

* **Cautions:** Start slow and build up. You can't bench press 300 pounds the first time you go to the gym. Trying to lift your legs as high as you can only *strains* your lower back.

* **Other Benefits:** Strengthens large muscles of the back and buttocks as well as the muscles that support the sacroiliac joint.

Vimanasana (*vimana* = chariot of the gods) means airplane posture. The next set of asanas is done lying on your belly with an ***inward hip rotation***. That means you are lying on the tops of your thighs, not the inside of your thighs.

Rest your chest and one cheek on the mat. Place your arms however they are comfortable. Try your forearms on the floor or your arms back by your sides.

There are three versions of leg lifts with ***increasing amounts of difficulty***.

A. Lifting one leg at a time.

LOWER BACK—SACROILIAC FIG. # 4

Exhale   *Inhale*

- As you inhale, lift one leg a few (two or three) inches off the floor. No need to go any higher.

- As you exhale, lower the leg to the floor.

- Inhale and lift the other leg, exhale and lower it.

- Repeat three to five times.

Tomorrow repeat five to seven times.

B. Lifting both legs together.

LOWER BACK—SACROILIAC FIG. # 5

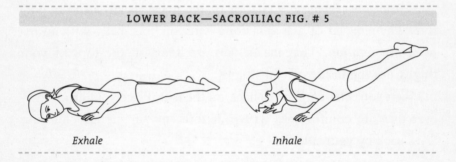

Exhale   Inhale

Begin with lifting both legs one to three times. Slowly, taking a few days, work up to ten times.

C. Lifting both legs and opening them as wide as you can.
Now you are ready to lift both legs—open them on inhale, then close on exhale and lower your legs to the floor. Trying to do too much too soon can easily cause more problems than you want. Take it easy and soon you will have a very strong and stable lower back.

LOWER BACK—SACROILIAC FIG. # 6

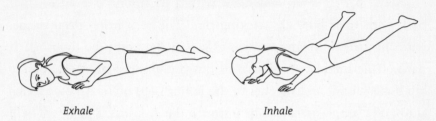

Exhale   Inhale

Please believe that the last version is much harder than it looks. This is truly an example of starting with a lower weight and working up progressively. With an *inward rotation* at the hips, the leg lift places a lot of the work in muscles in the lumbar/sacroiliac area. Some of the lifting will of course be done by your gluteus, but not as much as with an outward rotation. Thus, this is the exercise to strengthen your lumbar and sacroiliac area muscles.

Another technique is to build your leg lifts in "sets." An example would be to lift one leg three times then the other leg three times. Tomorrow, do the same thing twice or two "sets" of leg lifts three times each. When you increase the number of leg lifts, decrease the number of "sets." Work up to three "sets" or number of times you lift your legs three times each. The next day, lift each leg five times, but only do two "sets." When you increase the number of leg lifts, decrease the number of sets and work your way back up to three "sets" of leg lifts each day.

After whatever version of the leg lifts you are doing, immediately push up to your hands and knees and repeat *cakravakasana* (see page 29). Exhale and move your buttocks toward your heels as you fold forward. Repeat four or five times.

* * *

Some people walk and stand with a pronounced sway in their back with their buttocks sticking out. The reason lies deep inside, with the largest, longest muscle group in the body, the iliopsoas. It starts at the lumbar vertebra, runs down along the front side of the hip bone (ilium) and attaches to the femur (leg) bone. An easy adaptation of a simple asana can help stretch the iliopsoas, which will help relieve compression in the lower back and bring relief to the pelvic/sacrum/lumbar spine area.

EKAPADA USTRASANA VARIATION

* **Keep in Mind:** Keep your torso erect. The sink comes at the hips, not by leaning forward. Some people may need a little more padding under the back knee.

* **Cautions:** Keep your lower back long. Do not compress or collapse in the lumbar spine.

* **Other Benefits:** Also stretches quadriceps and increases hip mobility.

LOWER BACK—SACROILIAC FIG. # 7

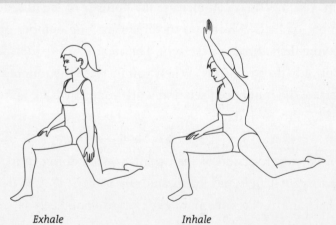

Exhale   Inhale

EKAPADA USTRASANA (EKA ONE, *PADA*-FOOT; *USTRA*-CAMEL) IS A ONE FOOT CAMEL POSTURE.

• Start with one leg back and your knee on the floor. Try to have the leg straight behind you with the top of the foot on the floor. Bring the other leg forward, knee bent, foot on the floor. Place your palms on the top of each of your thighs.

• Inhale, sink into the lunge, lift the hand resting on the back thigh, and push up with the heel of the hand.

• To protect the front knee, keep the front foot far enough forward so that as you sink into the lunge, the front knee should not come past the toes on that foot.

• Exhale and return to the start position.

• Repeat two times.

The second time, stay in the lunge with your arm up and take two deep breaths, each time pushing up harder with the heel of the hand. Feel the stretch deep on that side. Return to the start position.

Kneel on your mat. You will probably feel longer or taller on the side you stretched. Repeat other side.

SUPTA PADANGUSTHASANA

* **Keep in Mind:** If your legs do not straighten, it is okay to keep your knees slightly bent. Move with your breath.

* **Cautions:** Be aware of your lower back and the sacroiliac joint. If this is a strain, keep your knees bent. You will still receive much benefit.

* **Other Benefits:** Stretches hamstrings, groin muscles, and opens the hips.

LOWER BACK—SACROILIAC FIG. # 8

Exhale   Inhale   Exhale

Lie on your back, knees bent, feet up, and one hand behind each knee.

- Inhale, straighten both legs.

- Exhale, open your legs.

- Inhale, bring your feet back together.

- Exhale, bend your knees.

Repeat three or four times. After this movement becomes comfortable (two or three days, weeks, or months), stay in the open legs position for a few breaths.

APANASANA

Repeat *apanasana* (see page 44) three or four times, and then hug your thighs to your chest for a few breaths.

SAVASANA

Lie back on your yoga mat for *savasana*.

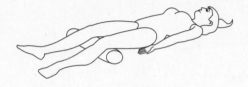

Place a rolled blanket under your knees to lengthen your lumbar spine. Close your eyes and once again breathe into your lower back for a few minutes. Visualize a strong, stable lower back.

By using the asanas in this chapter to lengthen my iliopsoas and stabilize my sacroiliac joint, I live a happy life. Also, I utilized this sequence for a student who had suffered lower back pain for more than a decade. Two weeks later, at the beginning of our second session, he was smiling. He said he had forgotten what life was like without pain. A strong, stable, supple lower back can be yours, too.

YOUR COMPLETE LOWER BACK—
SACROILIAC SEQUENCE

*   *   *

Breathing Guidelines

Inhale and exhale through your nose. * Remember to practice ujjayi breathing (control of the breath in the throat). * **On inhale, fill from the top to the bottom.** * As you exhale, empty from the bottom to the top by gently pulling in below the navel. * **Coordinate breathing and moving. Your breath is longer than the movement.** * It starts before the movement and finishes after the movement is completed. *

Start ←------------------BREATH------------------→ Finish

Start ←-----------MOVEMENT-----------→ Finish

See page 4 for details.

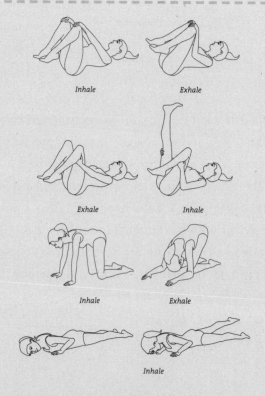

Inhale   Exhale

Exhale   Inhale

Inhale   Exhale

Inhale

continued

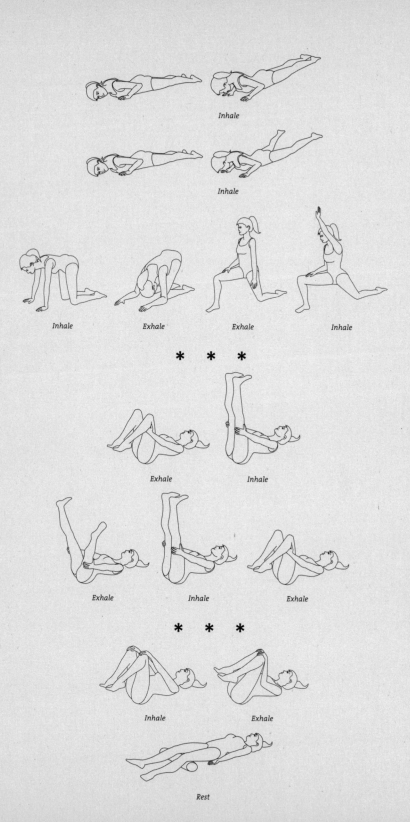

Inhale

Inhale

Inhale   *Exhale*   *Exhale*   *Inhale*

* * *

Exhale   *Inhale*

Exhale   *Inhale*   *Exhale*

* * *

Inhale   *Exhale*

Rest

Back Flexibility for Athletes

Do you play golf or tennis? Do you bowl, play softball, or play basketball? Back flexibility and strength enhances your performance in every sport. For example, a golfer twists his or her back 75 to 100 times in the same direction per round of golf. Do they ever think to twist in the other direction? How many golfers or tennis players take the time to do an easy forward bend to "neutral out" their lower back before, after, or during the game? Do you know a golfer with lower back or sacrum discomfort? I know many of them. Sacrum instability is the golfer's curse. It also inflects pain upon tennis, bowling, and softball enthusiasts. The previous two chapters showed you how to establish strength and stability in the lower back and sacroiliac. This chapter addresses shoulder and back flexibility. Would you like to be able to play golf or tennis forever? When you create and maintain a supple, fluid body, you open the door to longevity in your sports career. It could easily last into your seventies and eighties.

Would you like to easily turn your shoulders a little farther without twisting your hips and drop a few strokes or win a match point simply by increasing the mobility in your upper back? This is the chapter for you.

My friend Russell is a natural athlete. He is big, fast, and agile. Russell has played golf most of his life. He says that after he turned fifty, he actually got stronger and hit his drives longer. However, his shoulders and lower back became stiffer and tighter as he moved toward sixty. We set about to design a short flexibility program to increase his mobility and decrease the last number on his scorecard.

Seated Forward Bend

* **Keep in Mind:** Start your exhale by pulling in below the navel. To return to the upright position, inhale and lift your chest to come up with a flat back.

* **Cautions:** Avoid lifting your chin on inhale.

* **Other Benefits:** Strengthens as well as stretches lower back muscles.

Begin by sitting and connecting with your breath. Then "breathe" into your lower back. Take your breath and attention into the muscles in the lumbar area.

The first asana is a forward bend to stretch your lower back and prepare the lumbar area for the twists.

BACK FLEXIBILITY FIG. # 1

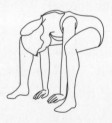

Exhale

- Sit forward on your chair. Exhale by gently pulling in below the navel and slide your hands down your legs toward the floor. Drop your chin to your chest and move your torso down between your thighs. Have your legs far enough apart to allow your chest to drop as far as it can. Stay for one breath.

- To come up, inhale, lift your chest (not your chin) slide your hands up your legs, and return to an upright sitting position. Repeat two times.

Seated Twists

* **Keep in Mind:** Move with your breath. *Remember, Exhale* and *Twist, Inhale* and *Unwind.*

* **Cautions:** Keep neck long—neither lift nor drop the chin.

* **Other Benefits:** Increased suppleness in cervical and thoracic spine.

BACK FLEXIBILITY FIG. # 2

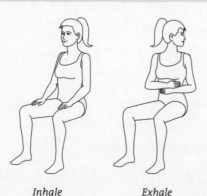

Inhale   Exhale

- Inhale and sit tall in your chair.

- Exhale, pull in below the navel, and twist.

Start the twist low in your back, not with the shoulder movement. Twist your entire torso, not just your shoulders and chin.

- Hold the twist for one breath; then, on your next inhale, unwind, returning to a neutral position.

- Exhale, twist the other direction, and hold the twist for one breath.

- Unwind on inhale.

- Repeat each side, holding for two breaths.

- Repeat each side again, holding for three breaths.

- To balance out, repeat the forward bend and hold for a few breaths.

These twists and the forward bend can be done sitting in a chair, on a bench next to the playing field, or on the seat of your golf cart.

Standing Shoulder Opener

* **Keep in Mind:** When sweeping your arms, push your fingertips away to straighten the arms and open the shoulders. Start your exhale by gently pulling in below your navel.

* **Cautions:** Do not force your arms to move farther than your shoulders will allow at first.

* **Other Benefits:** Increased mobility in shoulders.

• Stand up on your yoga mat with your feet flat on the floor. Bring your palms together in front of your chest.

• Keeping your elbows down, inhale, notice your breast bone lift as you inhale, and open your forearms as far as you comfortably can without compressing your lower back or lifting your chin. Come to a full stop with your movement and then your breath.

• Keeping the lift at the sternum, exhale and close your arms, bringing your palms back together.

BACK FLEXIBILITY FIG. # 3

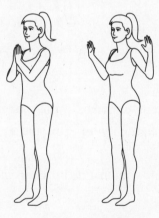

Inhale

• With your next inhale, sweep and straighten your arms out to the side and up over your head. Come to a full stop.

• Exhale and lower your arms, this time taking your hands behind you, turning your palms up, and feeling the arm bones (humerus) rotate in your shoulder; then, rest the backs of your hands in the lower back area.

BACK FLEXIBILITY FIG. # 4

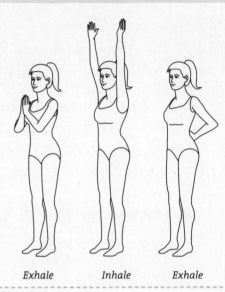

Exhale   Inhale   Exhale

When you sweep your arms, push your fingertips away from you to lengthen and straighten your arms and to open your shoulders.

• Inhale, sweep your hands up over your head, and come to a full stop.

• Exhale, lower your arms, and bring your palms together in front of your chest. This is the start position.

* * *

This Vinyasa (samasthiti to uttanasana) stretches and strengthens the lower back muscles.

The most important bit of information to remember is that ***bending your knees*** is the ***safety valve*** for your lower back. When you fold forward, let your knees **bend** slightly, also. Keep your knees **slightly bent** until you are all the way back up to the standing position. The movement creates much less strain in the lower back muscles with the **knees bent.** Thus, this repetition is much more beneficial with your **knees bent**, especially to the beginning practitioner.

Also, let's revisit the idea of arm placement to add or subtract weight to what is being lifted. The illustration instructs you to hold your arms up by your ears as you bend forward and as you lift back up to the standing position. This is the **most challenging**. You may want to start by bending forward and sliding your hands down the backs of your legs, and coming up by lifting your chest and sliding your hands up the backs of your legs. This is the least amount of weight your lower back has to carry.

Sweeping the arms to the side adds the weight of the arms, and holding your arms up by your ears adds both weight and length to the load. Please start slowly with two or three repetitions without using your arms. If that seems very easy on your lower back, tomorrow do two or three more, sweeping your arms out to the side as you bend forward and as you come up. Get some experience under your belt of how your lower back reacts before moving on to holding your arms by your ears. After you have built up some strength and flexibility in your lower back, it will be no big deal.

SAMASTHITI TO UTTANASANA

* **Keep in Mind:** Start your exhale by pulling in below the navel. To return to the standing position, inhale and lift your chest to come up with a flat back.

* **Cautions:** Avoid lifting your chin on inhale.

* **Other Benefits:** Stretches hamstring muscles.

BACK FLEXIBILITY FIG. # 5

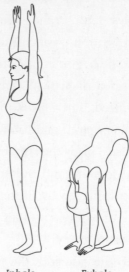

Inhale   *Exhale*

• Stand on your yoga mat. Have your feet hip-distance apart or wide enough to keep your balance as you bend forward and come up.

• Inhale, stand tall, and don't lift your arms the first time you try this posture. Instead, put your hands on your buttocks.

• Exhale, gently pull in below the navel, and fold forward (leading with your heart, not your chin), then **bend your knees** slightly and slide your hands down the back of your legs.

• To return to the standing position, inhale, lift your chest up and away from your thighs, and slide your hands up the back of your legs.

UTTANASANA WITH ARMS

• Stand with feet hip-distance apart. Inhale; sweep your arms out to the side and over your head.

• Exhale; pull in below the navel and fold forward, **bending the knees** slightly as you sweep your arms down. **Bend your knees** enough to touch the floor with your fingers.

• Keep the **bend in your knees**, inhale, and lift your chest as you sweep your arms to the side. Return to the standing position, lifting your arms over your head.

• Exhale and lower your arms to your side.

After you have practiced these first two versions for awhile, try it with your arms coming forward rather than out to the side. Always bend your knees. Go slow!

PARIVRTTI TRIKONASANA

*   **Keep in Mind:** Initiate both the forward bend and the twist below the navel.

*   **Cautions:** *Keep knees slightly bent* to protect your lower back. Keep your neck relaxed.

*   **Other Benefits:** Stretches lower back muscles and hamstrings.

Next, we will combine standing, forward bending, and twisting all at once in *parivrtti trikonasana* (twisting triangle pose). Stand with your feet wider than your hips or wide enough to create an equilateral triangle with your legs. That is, your feet are as far apart as your legs are long. There are three degrees of twisting in this sequence. Notice the "hash marks" in the drawing by the feet.

BACK FLEXIBILITY FIG. # 6

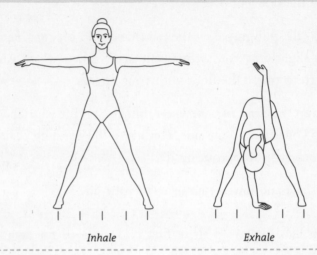

Inhale   Exhale

- Inhale, and lift your arms to the side at shoulder height.

- Exhale by pulling in below the navel; **bend your knees** slightly as you fold forward to touch the floor with your right hand between your feet. Stay and take one breath.

You can touch the floor with your fingertips or, if this is easy for you, put the palm of your hand on the floor. Nevertheless, **bend your knees** enough to touch the floor. Keep your neck relaxed; look down at your hand on the floor while lifting your left hand to point the fingers to the ceiling.

- Inhale, lift your chest, and return to the start position.

- Do the same thing with the other hand.

Next time, take your right hand *halfway* toward your left foot. Stay down for two breaths. Do the same thing with the left hand going *halfway* toward your right foot.

The last twist takes your hands as far as they will reach toward the opposite foot. Hold the twist for three breaths then come up, lower your arms, stand, and breathe.

UTTANASANA

Now do an easy forward bend as a counterpose to the twist.

Stand with your feet shoulder-width apart. **Bend your knees**, inhale, and put your hands on your buttocks. Exhale, fold forward, and slide your hands down the backs of your legs. Hang forward to stretch your lower back for a few breaths. To come up, keep your **knees bent**, inhale, and lift your sternum to come up with a flat back while sliding your hands up the backs of your legs.

BACK FLEXIBILITY FIG. # 7

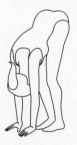

Exhale

---

*   *   *

Come on to your hands and knees in *cakravakasana* (see page 29). Exhale, and move your buttocks toward your heels as you fold forward. Repeat four or five times.

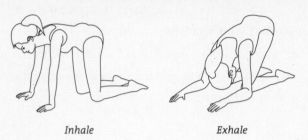

Inhale   *Exhale*

* * *

Sit and breathe. If you are a golfer, listen for the sound of the ball dropping into the cup. As you well know, if you peek, you pay. Or, try visualization. A bowler would "see" his ball hitting the pocket. The tennis player would "see" an ace serve. The softballer might hear the bat hitting the ball, knowing he hit the sweet spot and the ball is on its way out of the park.

In his book, *Golf My Way*, Jack Nicklaus reveals how he used visualization to become one of the greatest golfers of all time. Beforehand, he creates a mental movie of the entire golf shot in his head. He says he never hit a shot, even in practice, without this color movie. First he "sees" the ball where he wants it to finish, nice and white and sitting up high on the bright green grass. Then the scene quickly changes and he "sees" the ball going there: its path, trajectory, and shape, even its behavior on landing. Then there is a sort of fade-out, and the next scene shows him making the kind of swing that will turn the previous images into reality. See yourself at your best.

These asanas will take strokes off each round or add points to your batting average and add years of pain-free pleasure to your game. The simple twisting, arm movements and forward bends are custom-made for athletes.

YOUR COMPLETE BACK FLEXIBILITY SEQUENCE

* * *

Breathing Guidelines

Inhale and exhale through your nose. * Remember to practice ujjayi breathing (control of the breath in the throat). * **On inhale, fill from the top to the bottom.** * As you exhale, empty from the bottom to the top by gently pulling in below the navel. * **Coordinate breathing and moving. Your breath is longer than the movement.** * It starts before the movement and finishes after the movement is completed.

Start ◄------------------- B R E A T H ------------------→ Finish

Start ◄----------- M O V E M E N T ----------→ Finish

See page 4 for details.

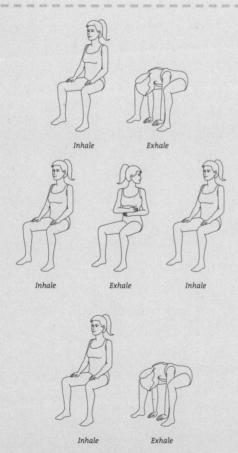

Inhale   Exhale

Inhale   Exhale   Inhale

Inhale   Exhale

continued

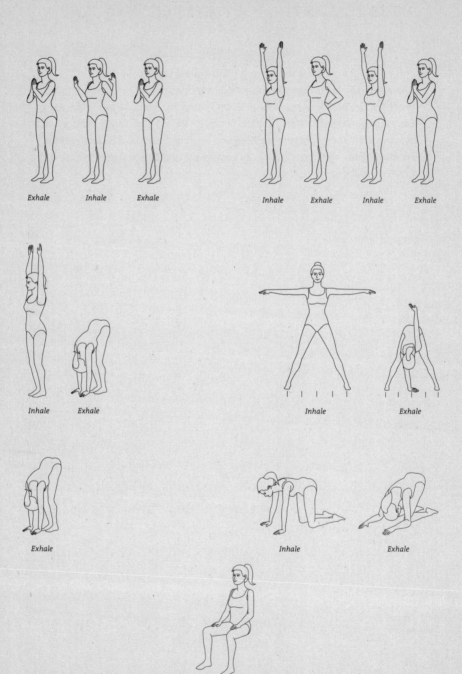

Exhale   Inhale   Exhale   Inhale   Exhale   Inhale   Exhale

Inhale   Exhale   Inhale   Exhale

Exhale   Inhale   Exhale

10

Constipation

Regularity is a blessing from heaven. Those who don't know that have never suffered from the problem of constipation. It can happen to anyone, but it seems to happen to the same people over and over. *Ayurveda*, the ancient medical system of India, classifies bodies in one of three types: *vata, pitta,* and *kapha.* Interestingly enough, constipation is often a near chronic affliction of people with a thinner (vata) body type rather than a medium (pitta) or thicker (kapha). For any of us, an upset stomach could lead to constipation. Anxiety can also manifest as poor elimination. What you ate yesterday may stay with you all day today. Whatever the cause, here is the cure.

A moderate sequence of twists and forward bends done standing, seated in a chair, and lying down will massage the lower intestinal area and greatly facilitate movement. Also, proper use of your breath will increase blood and energy flow and encourage relief.

Sit and breathe. Take your attention to your abdominal area. Feel the rise of your belly toward the end of your inhale. Start your exhale by slightly pulling in below the navel. See page 2 for the Basic Breathing Cycle. Breathe for thirty to sixty seconds and then start your asana practice.

VAJRASANA

* **Keep in Mind:** Push the tops of your feet into the floor for balance while bending forward and coming up. Push your fingertips away to straighten your arms and open your shoulders. To come up, lift your chest, not your chin.

* **Cautions:** If you cannot keep your balance bending forward while kneeling, or if kneeling is uncomfortable, do this asana in a chair for a while.

* **Other Benefits:** Lower back stretching and strengthening.

The first asana position, *vajrasana* (*vajra* = diamond, kneel, spine) is optional, depending on the condition of your knees. If you have already successfully tried kneeling and folding forward in the headache chapter, you will do a variation here. If this asana is too uncomfortable for your knees or back, try it sitting in a chair.

Kneel on your yoga mat. If you need more padding under your knees to be comfortable, place a folded blanket or towel on top of your yoga mat. Have enough padding under your knees to be comfortable but not so much that you are wobbly. Press the tops of your feet into the floor for balance. Place your hands, palms up, in your lower back or by your sides.

Inhale, lengthen your spine, and sweep your arms up over your head.

Start your exhale by pulling in with your lower abdominal muscles. As you fold forward, sweep your arms behind you, turn your palms up, turn your chin toward one shoulder, and take the side of your head toward the floor. Some of you will easily touch your head to the floor, while others will not get close. Don't worry about putting your head on the floor. The purpose of this exercise is to fold forward, not touch the floor or sit on your heels. Do not sit down— simply fold forward and stop when your body stops. You have already accomplished the purpose, which is massaging your stomach and intestines. If it is extremely awkward kneeling and bending forward, then sit in a chair (without arms) and follow the same instructions.

To come up, press the tops of your feet into the floor to maintain your balance. Start your inhale, lift your sternum (to come up with a flat back) while sweeping your arms out to the side and then over your head as you come upright.

CONSTIPATION FIG. # 1

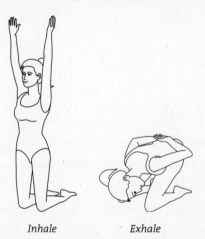

Inhale   Exhale

Start your exhale by pulling in with your lower abdominal muscles. Sweep your arms behind you; turn your chin the other direction while folding forward. Inhale, lift your chest, sweep your arms out to the side (pushing your fingertips away from you), and return to kneeling. Repeat three or four times.

Please don't overdo it when you first start practicing. All of these sequences require a slow buildup.

*   *   *

Come onto your hands and knees in *cakravakasana* (see page 29). Exhale, then move your buttocks toward your heels as you fold forward. Repeat four or five times.

CONSTIPATION FIG. # 2

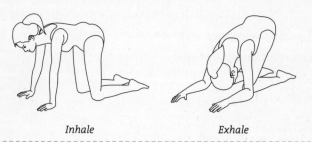

Inhale   *Exhale*

*   *   *

SAMASTHITI TO UTTANASANA

You may have already used these asanas in the Back chapters. The movements are the same, but ***you will change how you breathe to change the emphasis in your body***.

The most important bit of information to remember is that *bending your knees* is the ***safety valve*** for your lower back. Start folding forward, then let your knees bend slightly also. Keep your knees slightly bent until you are all the way back up to the standing position. The movement creates much less strain in the lower back muscles with the knees bent. Thus, this repetition is much more beneficial with your knees bent, especially to the beginning practitioner.

Also, let's revisit the idea of arm placement to add or subtract weight to what is being lifted. The illustration instructs you to hold your arms up by your ears as you bend forward and as you lift back up to the standing position. This is the **most challenging position**. You may want to start by bending forward and sliding your hands down the backs of your legs, and coming up by lifting your chest and sliding your hands up the backs of your legs. This is the least amount of weight your lower back has to carry.

Next time, try sweeping your arms to the side, which adds the weight of the arms. Holding your arms by your ears adds weight and length to the load. Please start slowly with two or three repetitions without using your arms. If that seems very easy on your lower back, tomorrow sweep your arms two or three more times. Get some experience under your belt of how your lower back reacts before moving on to holding your arms by your ears. After you have built up some strength and flexibility in your lower back, it will be no big deal.

Be careful—the instructions here are to hold your arms by your ears and repeat four times on the *hold after exhale*. When first practicing the asana, place your arms wherever they are comfortable for your back. The point of doing this is to massage your stomach and intestinal tract.

CONSTIPATION FIG. # 3

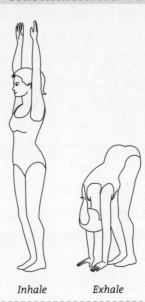

Inhale   Exhale

* **Keep in Mind:** Start your exhale by pulling in below the navel and *exhale completely*. To return to the standing position, inhale and lift your chest to come up with a flat back.

* **Cautions:** Avoid lifting your chin on inhale.

* **Other Benefits:** Stretches hamstring muscles.

• Stand on your yoga mat. Have your feet hip-distance apart or wide enough to keep your balance as you bend forward and come up.

• Inhale, stand tall, and do not lift your arms the first time you try this posture. Instead, put your hands on your buttocks.

• Exhale, gently pull in below the navel, and *exhale completely*. Then fold forward, leading with your heart (not your chin), bend your knees slightly, and slide your hands down the backs of your legs.

• To return to the standing position, inhale, lift your chest up and away from your thighs, and slide your hands up the backs of your legs. Repeat four times.

UTTANASANA WITH ARMS

• Stand with your feet hip-distance apart. Inhale; sweep your arms out to the side and over your head.

• Exhale; pull in below the navel and *exhale completely.* Then fold forward, bending the knees slightly as you sweep your arms down. Bend your knees enough to touch the floor with your fingers.

• Keep the bend in your knees, inhale, and lift your chest as you sweep your arms to the side. Return to the standing position, lifting your arms over your head.

• Exhale, and lower your arms to your side.

After you have practiced these first two versions for a while, try it with your arms coming forward rather than out to the side. Always bend your knees. Go slow!

PARIVRTTI TRIKONASANA

* **Keep in Mind:** Initiate both the forward bend and the twist below the navel. While holding after exhale, contract lower abdominal muscles a little more.

* **Cautions:** Keep knees slightly bent to protect your lower back. Keep neck relaxed.

* **Other Benefits:** Stretches lower back muscles and hamstrings.

Now a little twisting for the intestinal tract with *Parivrtti trikonasana* (twisting triangle pose) These asanas were used in the Back Flexibility for Athletes chapter to stretch the lower back muscles. Here they are used to massage and energize the stomach and intestines. Stand with your feet wider than your hips or wide enough to create an equilateral triangle with your legs. That is, your feet are as far apart as your legs are long. There are three degrees of twisting in this sequence. Notice the "hash marks" at the feet in the drawing.

CONSTIPATION FIG. # 4

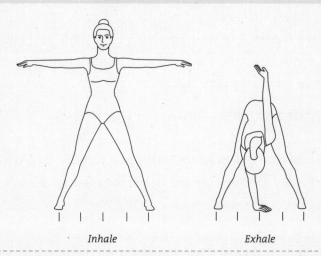

Inhale   Exhale

• Inhale; lift your arms to the side at shoulder height.

• Exhale by pulling in below the navel; bend your knees slightly as you fold forward to touch the floor with your right hand between your feet. Stay and take one breath, then **hold after the exhale for a count of two**.

You can touch the floor with your fingertips or, if this is easy, put the palm of your hand on the floor. Nevertheless, bend your knees enough to touch the floor. Keep your neck relaxed; look down at your hand on the floor while lifting your left hand to point your fingers to the ceiling.

- Inhale, lift your chest, and return to the start position.

- Do the same thing with the other hand.

Next time, take your right hand *halfway* toward your left foot. Stay down for a breath, then **hold after the exhale for a count of three.** Do the same thing with the left hand going *halfway* toward your left foot.

The last twist takes your hands as far as they will reach toward the opposite foot. Again, **hold the twist after exhale for a count of three**, then come up, lower your arms, stand, and breathe.

*   *   *

Come onto your hands and knees in *cakravakasana* (see page 29). Exhale and move your buttocks toward your heels as you fold forward. Repeat four or five times.

*   *   *

JATHARA PARIVRTTI

* **Keep in Mind:** Start slow, be easy on yourself. This asana is about twisting your belly, not about getting your knee to the floor.

* **Cautions:** Do not push your knee to the floor, as it may be too much for your lower back in the beginning.

* **Other Benefits:** Stretches lower back muscles.

CONSTIPATION FIG. # 5

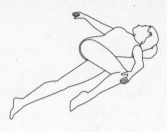

Exhale

- For *jathara parivrtti* (abdomen twist), lie on your back, arms out to the side, almost shoulder high, with your palms down. Lift your right foot and bend the right knee. Keep your foot up.

- As you exhale, twist your right knee toward the floor on the left side. Turn your chin to the right. Slightly lift your head off the floor (an inch or so) as you turn your chin in the opposite direction of the knee twist.

- On inhale, return to the start position. *This is twisting as you exhale.* Move with your breath. Start the exhale, then twist. Come to a full stop, then start the inhale and unwind. Repeat two or three times, then do the other side.

Next, from the start position, ***exhale completely*** and then twist. Do each side two or three times, each direction. *This is twisting* **after** *you exhale.*

The last stage of twisting is to exhale completely, twist one direction, and hold the twist for a few breaths. Then, twist to the other side and hold for a few breaths. When you finish, lie back with your feet on the floor and feel your belly. Take a few breaths before you move on.

SUPTA PADANGUSTHASANA VARIATION

∗ **Keep in Mind:** If your legs do not straighten, it is okay to keep your knees slightly bent. Move with your breath.

∗ **Cautions:** Be aware of your lower back and the sacroiliac joint. If this movement causes a strain, keep your knees bent. You will still receive much benefit.

∗ **Other Benefits:** Stretches groin muscles and opens the hips.

Lie on your back, knees bent and feet lifted off the floor. Put one hand behind each thigh to support your legs for the *supta padangusthasana* variation.

CONSTIPATION FIG. # 6

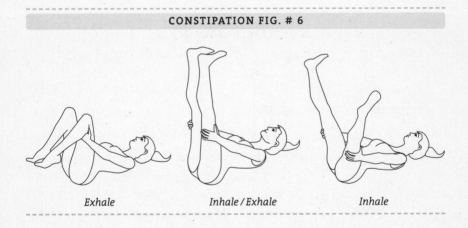

| Exhale | Inhale / Exhale | Inhale |

• Inhale; straighten both legs. Push your heels up toward the ceiling. Stay there as you exhale.

• On inhale, open your legs, taking your heels as far apart as they will comfortably go.

• Exhale; close your legs.

• Inhale; open your legs. Repeat two or three times, then close your legs and return to the start position with your knees bent.

If this is easy for you, stay in the open leg position for a couple of breaths; if not, don't. Repeat the whole thing one more time.

PASCIMATANASANA

* **Keep in Mind:** Keep knees bent and lengthen your spine as you fold forward.

* **Cautions:** Do not pull yourself farther forward with your arms.

* **Other Benefits:** Stretches and strengthens the lower back.

CONSTIPATION FIG. # 7

Inhale   *Exhale*

• Sit with your legs in front of you, *almost* straight, keeping a slight bend in the knees for *pascimatanasana* (stretching the back). As you inhale, lift your arms up over your head.

- As you exhale, fold forward, lowering your belly and chest toward your legs. Stay down and take **one** breath.

- Inhale; lift your arms and chest to come up with a flat back.

- Exhale, fold forward, and stay down for **two** breaths.

- Inhale; come up.

- Exhale, fold forward, and stay down for **three** breaths. Return to the start position and lower your arms.

Next, repeat this sequence, moving on the **hold after the exhale**. That is, inhale and lift your arms, stay up and **exhale completely, fold forward**, then take **one** breath.

Next time, fold forward while holding your breath after the exhale and stay down for **two** breaths.

The last time, stay down for **three** breaths. Return to the start position and lower your arms.

SAVASANA

CONSTIPATION FIG. # 8

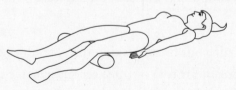

Rest

Lie back in savasana for a few minutes then sit up for the most important part of this sequence, *pranayama krama* (segmented breathing).

PRANAYAMA KRAMA

* **Keep in Mind:** Breathe slower rather than faster.

* **Cautions:** Do not overdo it in the beginning. Less is more.

* **Other Benefits:** Increasing your breathing cycle and your ability to hold your breath will greatly benefit all of your body systems.

If you are comfortable on your yoga mat, stay there. You can use a folded blanket or towel under your sitting bones for more comfort or sit in a chair.

• Inhale completely.

• Start the exhale by gently contracting below the navel. Exhale only half the breath, stop and hold your breath for two or three seconds, then exhale the rest of your breath, finishing the exhale by gently contracting above the navel. Hold your breath out for two or three seconds.

• As you inhale, try to release your muscles as your breath moves down. (See Basic Breathing Cycle, page 2.) First, release your upper abdominal muscles, then release your lower abdominal muscles.

• Exhale half your breath, taking three or four seconds; stop and hold your breath for two or three seconds; then exhale the second half of your breath, taking three or four seconds. Hold your breath out for three or four seconds. Repeat four or five times.

Slowly build up the amount of time that each segment of the exhale requires and how long you hold both between segments and at the end of the exhale. Work up to eight complete breaths. Also, work up to four or five seconds for each segment of the breath and the holding of the breath.

When you finish the krama breathing, sit quietly for a minute or two. Rearrange your sitting position if you are uncomfortable. Breathe easily. Place your hands on your abdomen, with one hand above the navel and the other below. Take your attention to your hands and then into your body. Use your breath and energy to soothe the area that has just been exercised. Daily repetition of this sequence brings daily regularity.

YOUR COMPLETE CONSTIPATION SEQUENCE

* * *

Breathing Guidelines

Inhale and exhale through your nose. ∗ Remember to practice ujjayi breathing (control of the breath in the throat). ∗ **On inhale, fill from the top to the bottom.** ∗ As you exhale, empty from the bottom to the top by gently pulling in below the navel. ∗ **Coordinate breathing and moving. Your breath is longer than the movement.** ∗ It starts before the movement and finishes after the movement is completed.

Start •-------------------BREATH-------------------→ Finish

Start •-----------MOVEMENT-----------→ Finish

See page 4 for details.

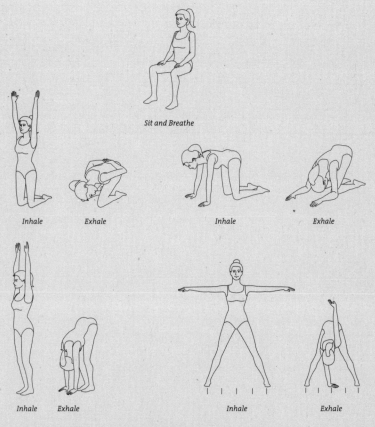

Sit and Breathe

Inhale   Exhale   Inhale   Exhale

Inhale   Exhale   Inhale   Exhale

continued

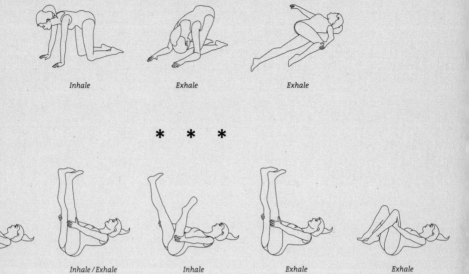

Inhale *Exhale* *Exhale*

* * *

Exhale *Inhale / Exhale* *Inhale* *Exhale* *Exhale*

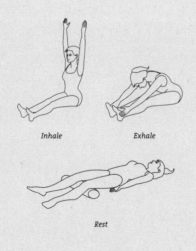

Inhale *Exhale*

Rest

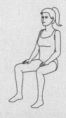

Krama breathing

11

Sexual Vigor

For men and women, normal, healthy sexual function is a some-times mysterious intertwining of physical, emotional, and psychological interplay. Take, for example, the conflict in time schedule between a woman's monthly ovulation cycle and the average man's semen cycle of four to eight times a month. It would seem to be a minor miracle that two people are ever "in the mood" on the same day. The physical aspects of the reproductive areas of the human body can be exercised to establish health and vitality. Specifically focusing on this area can greatly improve stamina, control, and sensitivity.

The breath is always important, but especially in this sequence using the Basic Breathing Cycle greatly increases the benefits. Revisit page 2 on Yoga Essentials for details.

While lying on the floor, we will start with a few simple asanas to exercise the muscle groups in the pelvic and groin area.

APANASANA

* **Keep in Mind:** Keep your shoulders on the floor. Keep your hands on your kneecaps. Coordinate breath and movement.

* **Cautions:** Don't pull too hard, this is a warm-up.

* **Other Benefits:** Will increase range of motion in hips.

Lie on your yoga mat. Bend your knees and lift your feet. Place one hand on each kneecap. As you exhale, gently but firmly pull your thighs toward your chest. Keep your hands on your kneecaps, inhale, and push your knees away.

SEXUAL VIGOR FIG. #1

Inhale   Exhale

Coordinate the movement with your breathing. Remember the short pauses that happen at the end of the exhale and the end of the inhale. That means start your exhale and then start pulling in. Finish the movement, finish the breath, and feel the short (half-second) pause. Then, start your inhale, straighten your arms, and come to a full stop. Repeat four or five times. A small pillow or a folded towel behind your head will make this position more comfortable. Focus your attention to your hips and think of breathing into them. Attention plus breath equals awareness. Awareness of what is happening in your body is half the battle. Awareness will ease your path to a supple, strong body.

SUPTA PADANGUSTHASANA VARIATION

* **Keep in Mind:** If your legs do not straighten, it is okay to keep your knees slightly bent. Move with your breath.

* **Cautions:** Be aware of your lower back and the sacroiliac joint. If this is a strain in your lower back, keep your knees bent. You will still receive much benefit.

* **Other Benefits:** Stretches groin muscles and opens the hips. Increases blood and energy flow to pelvic floor.

Lie on your back with knees bent and feet lifted off the floor. Put one hand behind each thigh to support your legs.

SEXUAL VIGOR FIG. # 2

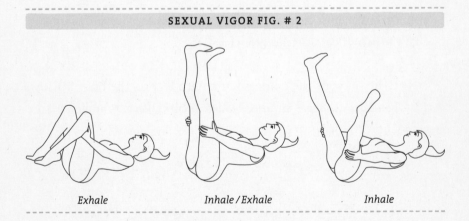

Exhale   Inhale / Exhale   Inhale

• Inhale; straighten both legs. Push your heels up toward the ceiling. Stay in this position as you exhale.

• On inhale, open your legs, taking your heels as far apart as they will comfortably go.

• Exhale, then close your legs.

• Inhale; open your legs. Repeat two or three times, then close your legs and return to the start position with your knees bent.

*   *   *

If this is easy for you, stay in the open leg position for a couple of breaths; if not, don't. Repeat the whole sequence one more time.

*   *   *

Repeat *apanasana* (see page 44).

SUPTA BADDHA KONASANA

* **Keep in Mind:** Move with your breath.

* **Cautions:** If this creates discomfort in your lower back, discontinue.

* **Other Benefits:** Increases hip mobility. Increases blood and energy flow to pelvic floor. Stretches groin muscles.

Next, lie on your back, knees bent, with feet on the floor for *supta baddha konasana* (*supta* = supine, *baddha* = bind, *kona* = angle).

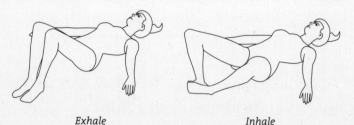

SEXUAL VIGOR FIG. # 3

Exhale   *Inhale*

- Inhale and open your knees.

- Exhale; close your knees. Repeat five or six times.

UPAVISTHA KONASANA ADAPTATION

* **Keep in Mind:** Begin each of your exhales by pulling in below your navel.

* **Cautions:** Do not pull yourself farther forward with your arms.

* **Other Benefits:** Stretches hamstrings and lower back. Increases hip mobility.

Sit up on your yoga mat for *upavistha konasana* adaptation (*up-avista* = to sit, *kona* = angle). Open your legs as far as they will comfortably go. Bend your knees.

SEXUAL VIGOR FIG. # 4

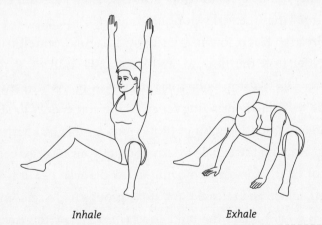

Inhale   *Exhale*

- Lift your arms alongside your ears and above your head as you inhale.

- Exhale; bend forward between your legs. Stay for one breath.

- Inhale, then lift your arms and your chest to come up with a flat back.

You may want to make an adjustment in your leg position. Keep them as wide as is comfortable. Try bending your knees a little more. Try it again. Inhale, lift your arms, exhale, then bend forward between your legs. Stay for a few breaths, then come up as you inhale. Try it one last time.

KRAMA-SEGMENTED BREATHING

The most beneficial element of this sequence is controlling the breath in conjunction with contracting and relaxing the abdominal muscles. The breathing exercise, krama-segmented breathing, will greatly increase muscle tone, the health of your vital organs, digestive system function, help reduce incontinence after pregnancy, and increase or reestablish sexual vigor.

Sit. Breathe. Relax low in your body. Imagine yourself to be urinating. Now stop the flow in mid-stream. Feel all of the muscle groups you used to stop your imaginary peeing. As you strengthen those muscles, you are bringing renewed life and energy to all of the sexual organs also. Exercising those muscles begins with proper breathing. Starting the exhale by contracting your muscles beginning at the floor of the torso and moving up to the *solar plexus* is the first step. Then, inhale and release the muscle groups in descending order.

As you inhale, retain the mild contraction below the navel while relaxing only from the *solar plexus* to the *navel*, pause, then continue the inhale and relax from the *navel* to the *pubic bone*, then from the *pubic bone* to the *floor of the torso*. At first, this muscle coordination seems impossible, but strength and control will improve with practice. All the while, you are building stronger muscles the same way lifting a dumbbell strengthens your biceps.

The next step is to exhale in stages while also contracting the muscles in stages.

- Start your exhale and gently contract the muscles from the *bottom of the torso* to the *pubic bone*. Pause.

- Continue your exhale and contract the muscles between the *pubic bone* and the *navel*. Pause.

- Finish your exhale while contracting the muscles from the *navel* to the *solar plexus*.

Now, inhale in segments.

- First, inhale and release the muscles from the *solar plexus* to the *navel* while retaining the gentle contractions below. Pause.

- Continue your inhale while releasing the muscle contraction from the *navel* to the *pubic bone*. Pause.

- Finish your inhalation and release the muscles from the *pubic bone* to the *floor of the pelvis*.

Do five complete breath cycles. Then, sit and breathe normally for a minute before you get up and move onto your next activity.

This krama breathing can also be used by itself. If you try it for just a minute or two in the morning, you will notice that it builds warmth and energy in the body. Or, try one round of krama breathing while waiting for a red traffic light to turn green. If you make this breathing technique part of your daily practice, very shortly you will notice increased muscle tone in your abdomen. Other results will also become apparent.

YOUR COMPLETE SEXUAL VIGOR SEQUENCE

* * *

Inhale   *Exhale*

* * *

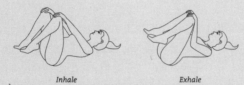

Exhale   *Inhale / Exhale*   *Inhale*   *Exhale*   *Exhale*

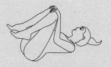

Inhale   *Exhale*

continued

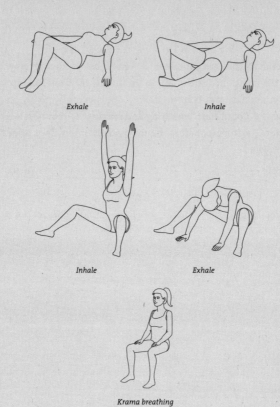

Exhale

Inhale

Inhale

Exhale

Krama breathing

12

The Brain

You can increase your memory, thinking power, perception, and concentration with *asana* and *pranayama*. Moving both sides of your body simultaneously (called opposition) causes both brain hemispheres to operate at the same time and creates a crossover function with the electrical brain messages, which in turn exercises the brain and makes it stronger and more supple.

After a recent conversation with a middle-aged friend, whose mother is declining deeper into Alzheimer's disease, I decided to start exercising my brain now and not to sit and wait for problems to emerge before taking action. It would be wise if we all assumed we had a very early, mild onset of memory loss. I think we should start doing something about it today. If you've got a brain and would like to keep it functioning at its best, this is the chapter for you.

BRAIN EXERCISE

Sit in a chair, feet flat on the floor, and your palms on your thighs. Concentrate on your inhale and exhale for a few seconds to connect with your breathing.

Inhale, lift one arm and the *opposite* foot, and then exhale as you lower them.

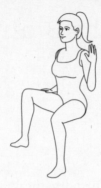

Inhale

Switch sides a few times. Lift on inhale and lower on exhale.

YOUR NECK

* **Keep in Mind:** Move with your breath. Stay within your comfortable range of motion.

* **Cautions:** Do not push yourself into pain.

* **Other Benefits:** Brings suppleness to thoracic and lumbar spine.

Next, do a sitting twist by moving your shoulders in one direction and your chin in the other direction.

Sit up. Relax your neck and your throat. Lengthen your neck but don't lift your chin. Let the top of your head float up as if there is a puppeteer's string attached that gently lengthens your neck. Inhale and, as you exhale, turn your chin to the *right*, but turn your shoulders to the *left*. Inhale, unwind, and return to neutral.

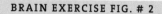

BRAIN EXERCISE FIG. # 2

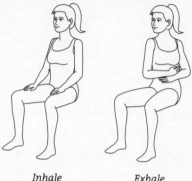

Inhale   *Exhale*

Your chin is moving one way and your shoulders are twisting the other direction. This opposition will not only give a good stretch to your neck, it will boost your brain power. Alternate sides and repeat four times. Twist on exhale and unwind on inhale.

CROSS CRAWLING

Come down onto all fours (hands and knees) on your yoga mat. Place your hands under your shoulders and your knees under your hips. You are going to walk forward using the opposite hand and knee, known as cross crawling. Take a "step" forward using your **right hand** and your **left knee**.

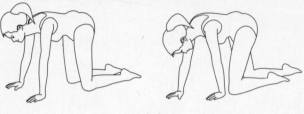

Inhale

Step again with your **left hand** and **right knee**. Take a few more steps. You may have to talk yourself through this the first time. Then, back up. "Step" back with one hand and the opposite knee. Walk back a few steps.

Go forward again. Back up again. Fun, isn't it? This exercise was used very successfully by people with attention-deficit disorder (ADD) before taking a test. It focuses the attention and balances the brain.

SUPTA PADANGUSTHA VARIATION

* **Keep in Mind:** Coordinate your breath with your movement. Start the breath, then start the movement. Start and finish straightening the leg and lifting the arm at the same time.

* **Cautions:** People with a Lumbar Disk That Is Currently "Bulging" Should Not Straighten Their Legs in This Position.

* **Other Benefits:** Balances body-mind interaction. Improves mental focus.

Lie on your back on the floor. Bend your knees, and lift your feet up off the floor with your arms at your side. Then, straighten one leg up toward the ceiling and lift the opposite arm up over your head, bringing your fingers to the floor behind your head. On exhale, return to the starting position. Do both sides and repeat four or five times.

BRAIN EXERCISE FIG. # 4

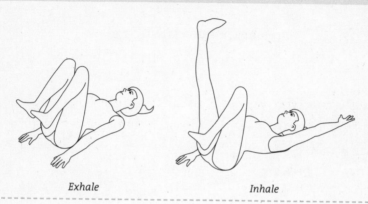

Exhale   Inhale

---

* * *

DVIPADA PITHAM VARIATION

* **Keep in Mind:** When you roll up, lengthen your neck by dropping your head and chin toward your sternum.

* **Cautions:** Keep your lower back long, not compressed.

* **Other Benefits:** Flexibility and suppleness in the spine.

You previously did an exercise called dvipada pitham, two-foot pose (see page 45). This time, we will change the arm movements to challenge your brain. While on your back, place your arms at your sides with your knees bent and feet flat on the floor about hip-distance apart. Place your heels under your knees. Inhale, push down with your feet, lift your hips off the floor, and raise your arms up over your head, then toward the floor behind you. As you exhale, lower your back along the floor and lower your arms down, bringing the palms back to the floor by your sides. Keep the tuck in your hips so that your lower back touches the floor before your buttocks do. On your next inhale, lift your hips and arms, but stop one arm as it points to the ceiling while continuing to move the other arm.

BRAIN EXERCISE FIG. # 5

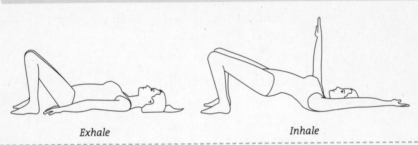

Exhale   *Inhale*

Exhale, then lower your back and the one arm that is over your head. When that arm reaches the same place as the arm that stopped, bring them both down together with your back. Roll up and down with your breath. Inhale up; exhale down. Alternate arms, stopping one arm when the fingers point to the ceiling, and repeat four or five times. When you finish, hug your knees toward your chest for a few breaths.

ARDHA SALABHASANA VARIATION

* **Keep in Mind:** Lift your chest, not your chin on inhale. Keep your neck long. Only lift your leg a few inches.

* **Cautions:** Keep your chin down; look down at your yoga mat in the up position.

* **Other Benefits:** Strengthens back muscles. Increases mobility in shoulders and neck.

Lie on your stomach with your arms at your sides or with your hands palms up in your lower back if that is easy on your shoulders. This is a repeat of *ardha salabhasana* but with an arm movement variation. As you inhale, you are going to lift one leg (just a few inches off the floor) and sweep one arm forward. Do not try to lift your leg as high as you can. That is counterproductive. If sweeping a straight arm causes discomfort, bend your elbow. See Tension Headache (page 32) for the illustration. It sounds complicated, but after a few times you will have it down pat.

BRAIN EXERCISE FIG. # 6

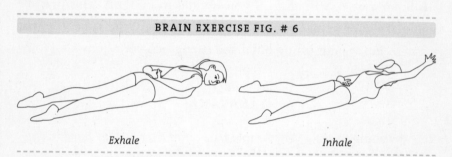

Exhale   Inhale

Now here's the tricky part—each time, the arm-leg combination will change. For example, the first time, lift your **right arm** and **right leg**. The second time, lift your **right arm** and **left leg**. Then, lift your **left arm** and **left leg**. Lastly, lift your **left arm** and **right leg**. You have now completed all of the possible combinations. Repeat the combinations, but go through the sequence starting with your left arm and left leg. Do all four possible combinations. It is difficult (on your mind, not your body). I had to slowly talk myself through each step of this sequence the first time I did it, but you will catch on with a little practice.

CAKRAVAKASANA

Come onto your hands and knees to cakravakasana (see page 29). Exhale, then move your buttocks toward your heels as you fold forward. Repeat four or five times. This asana is used as a counterpose to stretch and relieve tension in your lower back.

These asanas will do for your brain what going to the gym four times a week would do if you wanted to bulk up. This practice will make your brain stronger and more supple in the same way that exercise and weight lifting build and strengthen your body.

TADASANA

You are going to do a very simple balancing exercise, tadasana (tada = straight tree). Stand with your feet about hip-width apart. As you inhale, lift your heels off the floor, and as you exhale, lower your heels back to the floor. Some people can easily rise up onto the balls of their feet, while others will just lift their heels an inch or two off the floor. Either way, do it three or four times. Now stand on both feet and take a breath.

Next, inhale, and lift your heels and your arms out to the side and up over your head. Exhale; lower your arms and your heels. Repeat three or four times.

Now, inhale, and lift your heels and your arms, but stop your **left arm** when it reaches shoulder height and continue lifting the **right** arm up over your head. This is similar to the arm motion you did earlier in *dvipada pitham*.

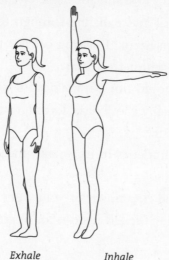

Exhale   *Inhale*

Exhale; lower your **right arm** to the level of your **left arm**, then lower them both as you lower your heels. This may not be much fun at first, but I promise you what it does for your brain you can't buy with money.

PRANAYAMA-NADI SODHANA

Lastly, sit and breathe to balance your system. The breathing technique for balance is alternate nostril breathing.

Do not skip this step. The power of breath is one of the most important tools at your disposal.

Nadi sodhana (*nadi* = passage way, *sodhana* = cleansing) is alternate nostril breathing that will help you balance your entire mind/body system.

The ancient masters teach that states of stimulation or relaxation can be regulated with control of the breath at the nostrils. Inhaling through the right nostril and exhaling through the left nostril will theoretically activate or stimulate your system, while inhaling through the left nostril and exhaling through the right nostril will soothe and calm your system. To bring balance to the system, combine both techniques with *nadi sodhana*.

This technique should not be practiced if your nostrils are obstructed or blocked in any way. Never force breath through your nostrils in *pranayama* practice.

There are many subtleties in *pranayama* practice. I will list a few of them for *nadi sodhana*.

Use the thumb and ring finger of your right hand. (In India and many Eastern countries, the left hand is for use in the bathroom.)

THE BRAIN FIG. #8

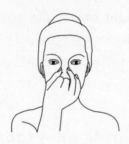

Do not use ujjayi breathing (control of the breath in the throat) when you are controlling the breath with the nostrils. Gently close your right nostril and inhale through your left nostril. Next, close your left nostril and exhale through your right nostril. Inhale through the right, close the right, then exhale through the left. That is one round of breathing. Keep both the thumb and ring finger in contact with your nose at all times. You will be able to feel the breath passing through the nostrils with your fingers. Close the nostril high on the nose, just below the hard cartilage at the bridge of the nose. You will be able to feel where the nostril closes. Start slow. Work with the breathing ratios in Yoga Essentials, page 4.

Yoga is holistic; it is not just asanas (the physical postures). Exercise your brain with new tasks (e.g., take a class or work puzzles). In June 2003, the *New England Journal of Medicine* reported that people who did crossword puzzles four days a week decreased their risk of dementia in half compared to subjects who did crossword puzzles once a week. Also, consider your diet—as much as you can, eat fresh, non-processed, chemical-free foods. All of these actions will result in a stronger mind.

. If you want to learn music and your and neighbors won't kill you, buy a drum kit. My friend Steve, the rock-and-roll drummer, uses both hands and both feet simultaneously, with each working independently and doing a different task. Or, to start slower, you can rub the top of your head while you pat your stomach. It all helps! If you are not doing puzzles or playing drums four times a week, start doing the exercises in this chapter to keep a healthy brain.

YOUR COMPLETE BRAIN SEQUENCE

* * *

Breathing Guidelines

Inhale and exhale through your nose. * Remember to practice ujjayi breathing (control of the breath in the throat). * **On inhale, fill from the top to the bottom.** * As you exhale, empty from the bottom to the top by gently pulling in below the navel. * **Coordinate breathing and moving. Your breath is longer than the movement.** * It starts before the movement and finishes after the movement is completed.

Start ●-------------------BREATH-------------------→ Finish

Start ●------------MOVEMENT----------→ Finish

See page 4 for details.

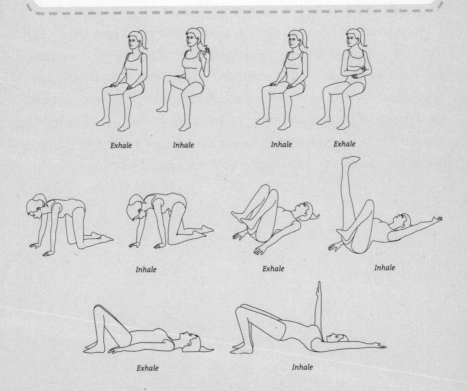

Exhale   Inhale   Inhale   Exhale

Inhale   Exhale   Inhale

Exhale   Inhale

continued

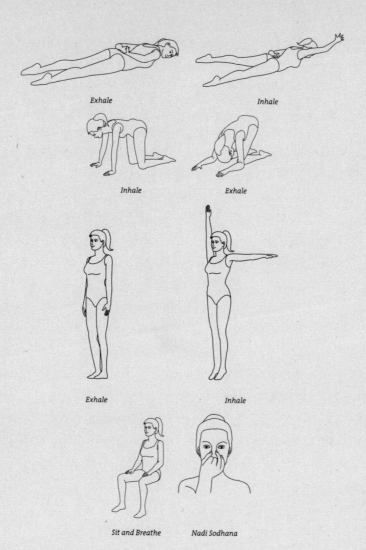

Exhale   Inhale

Inhale   Exhale

Exhale   Inhale

Sit and Breathe   Nadi Sodhana

13

Looking Within for Healing

Yoga can become more than postures and breathing. It can provide an opportunity for introspection that can help you to discover the deeper causes of aches, pains, and other troubles in your life. Additionally, you can deepen your practice by using it as a sacred ritual.

Svadhyaya

Is your lower back pain the result of weekend gardening or fear of your employer's impending downsizing? One person's tension headaches are another's back pain. In a third body, anxiety may manifest as poor elimination. Here the yogic concept of *svadhyaya* enters the picture. *Sva* means self and *adhyaya* translates as study or investigation. With self-investigation, you may find that when you're annoyed with your boss or spouse, your stomach becomes upset. An upset stomach could lead to constipation, which eventually may become colitis. Do you want to live with the pain? Will you get a new job or a divorce? The insight gained through your use of *svadhyaya* may give you a new perspective on the situation. You may feel able to initiate a conversation about the problem, where you may find some middle ground and seek a resolution.

There is no better time for self-examination than during your yoga practice. The ancient sages have a saying, "How you do anything is how you do everything." That means that your yoga practice is a mirror for the rest of your life. Think about how you are in your life. Does your mind wander? Is your breath short and choppy? Do you stop breathing altogether in situations of anxiety or apprehension? Your yoga practice will teach you how to breathe through difficult situations simply by breathing and continuing with your practice. It will improve the way you operate in your life. It will give you the opportunity to look at yourself from the inside out. You will learn something about your body and mind that you didn't know before.

When you finish your physical asana and pranayama practice, take a few extra moments for contemplation. Sit comfortably and quietly. Remind yourself of your main priorities and goals in life. What would you like to accomplish in your remaining years? What will be your legacy? What would you like to see as the epitaph on your tombstone? Your intuition or spirit will answer these questions for you when your mind and body are quiet and relaxed after your practice.

Pranayama—Breath

Throughout this book, I have suggested that you coordinate your movements with your breath. Paying attention to the movements of your body and breath with your mind creates awareness. Awareness keeps you in the present moment, the "Right Here—Right Now."

Not the past or the future, but now. You may already have noticed that your mind wanders and random thoughts distract you from your yoga session. The ability to concentrate is like a muscle. As you exercise it, your ability to concentrate will get stronger. That's the good news. The bad news is, it never gets perfect. However, this lack of perfection is part of the human condition.

Sacred Ritual

The goal of Viniyoga is to create the dual qualities of alertness and relaxation in all of life. One way for me to do that with exercise is to make it a sacred ritual that I like and want to do, rather than a penance or punishment that I have to do. By adding the use of affirmations, prayers, or mantras to my asana practice, I have deepened my experience. As I breathe, I repeat a few words that are holy or sacred to me. An example of such an affirmation is, "My mind is quiet and my heart is strong." I combine all aspects of myself—I move my body, coordinated with my breath, as I recite my favorite prayer or poem. Or I hold the thought and image of gratitude, grace, or my faith in God. Doing this anchors my personal spiritual beliefs in my heart and creates, among other things, emotional stability. The addition of ritual to one's physical practice opens the opportunity for the practitioner to reach a feeling of support and a sense of well-being.

Japa—Prayer/ Affirmation/Mantra

Over the years of teaching yoga, I have noticed that many asana students have very active minds. Many of us have a lot of mind chatter.

There is a yogic story that compares mind chatter to being like a drunken monkey, hyperactive and without direction.

The second of Patanjali's *Yoga Sutras* suggests that yoga can quiet the variations, chatter, or ripples of the active mind. One of the many exercises that Patanjali suggests, along with pranayama (breath) and asana, is *japa*. *Japa* is the repetition of a mantra that can be holy or sacred words.

Regarding what words to repeat, Patanjali refers us to the *pranavah*, which is the name of God. TKV Desikachar says that the *pranavah* is specific to each culture and religion. If you are a Hindu, it would possibly be OM. For a Muslim, the name of God is Allah. A Jew might say Adonoi Elohanu (A-do-noi El-o-ha-nu). A Christian could repeat the name of Jesus Christ. The point is, it's up to each person to decide what is holy and sacred to them. Think about what would be appropriate and desirable for you.

I believe it would be inappropriate for me as a yoga teacher to suggest a Sanskrit mantra to a practicing Muslim. Likewise, I would not pick a passage from the New Testament for an Orthodox Jew. Some people want nothing to do with the major religions. Their mantra might be a song, a poem, or something else that connects them to the Creative Force of the Universe.

One of my students had no religious or spiritual upbringing. There is no "conventional" image or set of words for him to use. I asked him where he saw God. He answered, "In the smile of my eight-year-old daughter." With those words he created a *bhavana*, a mental image, for himself. I suggested he try using the affirmation, "God, please help me to be the man my daughter thinks I am." Whether he believes in God or not, by using this phrase as his affirmation, he will experience a presence of that which is larger than himself in the universe, and he will manifest a desire to grow as a human being.

Your mantra is yours, not your teacher's. If you already have a favorite prayer or are currently using an affirmation, begin to incorporate it into your yoga practice. Let's say your affirmation is "I am healthy, wealthy, and wise." As you inhale, silently say your affirmation. As you exhale, silently repeat your affirmation.

At the end of this chapter, there are a few traditional prayers. You may find a short phrase that will get you started using words in your practice. Later you may settle on a different song, poem, or prayer.

Bhavana

Bhavana is an intention or a mental image. For some of you, it will be a religious image. For others, something more generic will be appropriate. If you have decided to add a small table to your practice area, place an image, picture, or symbol in front of you to inspire you throughout your yoga practice. I have experienced the presence of God in churches around the world, as well as while standing in Monument Valley, Utah. I used a photo I took there as the cover of my first book. I "see God" in photos by Ansel Adams and in paintings by Fredrick Church of the Hudson River school. Whatever images speak to your spirit—nature, art, architecture, family photographs—are appropriate for your space.

Nyasa

Nyasa means gesture. As you open and close your arms, repeat your affirmation and see your *bhavana*. Also, touch your chest or forehead and place the quality or energy of your *bhavana* and affirmation into your heart and mind.

I have found it very helpful to use a personal mantra to focus my mind. But this is not the only reason you would want to use a mantra. In the *Tibetan Book of Living and Dying*, it is recommended that we practice for the moment of our death. In their tradition, that moment determines our next incarnation, that is, do we return to earth for more lessons to be learned, or do we move upward into the sphere of the gods? We will live a happier, more productive, and peaceful life if each day we are already prepared for the moment of our last breath and thought.

Imagine for a moment that it is a dark and rainy night. You are driving on a mountain road. As you round a hairpin curve, you realize, too late, that your car is traveling too fast. In a heartbeat, you have crashed through the guardrail and are sailing into eternity. What is the thought in your mind? Oh, shit, or oh, God? What do you want your last thought to be?

Creating and using a personal mantra brings a multitude of benefits. One of them is that moment to moment during the day there is always something to refocus on when the drunken monkey is running wild in your head. Your personal mantra will become your new "default setting" that always pops up when needed.

Mantra can also be used as the doorway to meditation. In the morning or evening, after your asana practice, sit quietly and use *japa*, repetition of a prayer or affirmation, as the transition from the physical into the mental concentration portion of your yoga practice. Begin your meditation practice by repeating your personal mantra. That action will aim you in the direction you wish to go. It might be to merge with your God or whatever your goal may be.

For many of us, our childhood had religious overtones. Some of us were given a string of beads and a prayer to say over and over again for each one, as in the Catholic or Hindu faith. Others of us thumbed through books of scriptures, repeating page after page of prayers, as in the Jewish or Buddhist tradition. Whatever your childhood exposures were, saying prayers over and over at your current stage of life could become a form of relaxation. If you enjoyed it and did it because you wanted to, it may even lead to a mystical experience. The practice of repeating a set of words to calm down the emotions has been around for as long as there have been words to repeat. Its calming effect comes from using meaningful words as a point of focus.

Finding the Words

What set of words, if any, would you like to say over and over? What words bring you joy and guidance? A prayer from your youth, or perhaps a new one, such as the Prayer of St. Francis of Assisi or the "Serenity Prayer"? Notice that each of these prayers has short phrases that can easily be incorporated into your yoga practice. For example, you might use "May I seek to understand" from the prayer of St. Francis.

Or you may find words to suit you in other traditions. Here are a few examples and ideas you may use to begin with.

PRAYER OF ST. FRANCIS OF ASSISI

Lord, make me an instrument of Thy peace;
where there is hatred, let me sow love; / where there is injury, pardon; /
where there is doubt, faith; / where there is despair, hope;
where there is darkness, light; / and where there is sadness, joy.
　　O Divine Master,
　　grant that I may not so much
seek to be consoled, as to console; / to be understood, as to understand;
to be loved, as to love; / for it is in giving that we receive,

*it is in pardoning that we are pardoned, / and it is in dying that we are
born to eternal life.*

SHEMA

She-ma Yis-ra-el	*Hear, O Israel*
A-do-noi El-o-ha-nu	*the Lord our God*
A-do-noi Ech-had	*the Lord is One*

TIBETAN BUDDHIST MANTRA
Om Mani Padma Hum

THE SERENITY PRAYER
*God, grant me the serenity to
accept the things I cannot change,
the courage to change the things I can,
and the wisdom to know the difference.*

(© 1962 Reinhold Niebuhr, American theologian, 1892–1971)

A code of personal conduct is contained in the *Yoga Sutras*. The
guiding principles will be familiar to all, and any of these principles
can serve as a beginning affirmation. You might pick one word as a
quality you would like to have more of in your life.

THE *YAMAS*—OUR ACTIONS TOWARD OTHERS

1. *Consideration* toward all living things, especially those who are in-
nocent, in difficulty, or worse off than we are.
2. *Right communication* through speech, writings, gesture, and actions.
3. *Noncovetousness*, or the ability to resist a desire for that which does
not belong to us.
4. *Moderation* in all our action.
5. *Nongreediness*, or the ability to accept only what is appropriate.

THE *NIYAMAS*—OUR ACTIONS TOWARD OURSELVES

1. *Cleanliness*, or the keeping of our bodies and our surroundings clean and neat.

2. *Contentment*, or the ability to be comfortable with what we have and what we do not have.

3. The removal of impurities (*cleansing*) in our physical and mental systems through the maintenance of such correct habits as sleep, exercise, nutrition, work, and relaxation.

4. *Study* and the necessity to review and evaluate our progress.

5. *Reverence* to a higher intelligence, or the acceptance of our limitations in relation to God, the all-knowing.

This text is taken from Heart of Yoga, *TKV Desikachar,* Inner Traditions Intl. Ltd., 1999.

Or recite a favorite poem, such as Robert Frost's "Stopping by Woods on a Snowy Evening," which ends with a repetition of the line "And miles to go before I sleep." If you like to sing, begin chanting your most loved spiritual song, such as "Amazing Grace," which begins with the inspiring words "Amazing grace, how sweet the sound that saved a soul like me." When deciding on a poem or song to use as a point of focus, be sure to choose one that touches you. Then see what it does for your mind.

Remember, the techniques that suit the teacher may not suit the student, so don't be turned away by these particular examples. They are among my favorite poems and songs. Use those that stir your soul.

Sound (Chant/Sing)

Another way of working with words is to repeat them aloud or to chant them. An example would be to inhale and lift your arms up over your head. As you exhale, say the affirmation out loud and bring your palms together in front of your chest.

Now it's time to put some of these ideas into practice. Revisit the first sequence. Before you begin, decide on a thought, image, or set of words that will be your theme for today. Maybe you would like to place a picture of your family or a spiritual icon in front of you. Take a moment to see the image and breathe it into you. Then begin your practice.

14

Putting It All Together

Yoga, simply defined by TKV Desikachar, is the "ability to direct the mind exclusively toward an object and hold that direction without any distractions." What do you want to direct your mind toward? How about each moment as you live it? I call this being Right Here, Right Now. This could be your practice while you are doing it, your job as you perform it, and your interpersonal relationships as you actively participate in them. Altogether, it means your life, one heartbeat at a time.

The practice of yoga is holistic; it has positive effects on the entire human being, physical, emotional, and spiritual. Whether your goal is to relieve back pain or mental anxiety, yoga is the vehicle to carry you there. Viniyoga uses all of the tools of yoga to develop a personal practice including *tapas*, the physical and mental practice, to generate the heat and energy necessary for forward movement in your life; *svadyaya*, self-examination, to point the direction in which you want to move; and *ishvara pranidana*, devotion to a Higher Power, which provides the courage and faith to persevere on your journey. Through the use of your personal practice, you learn to improve the day-to-day quality of your life and tools to link you with your own Higher Power. Yoga is also a vehicle that will help you move along your chosen spiritual path.

Namaste. I honor the Spirit in you.

BIBLIOGRAPHY

Desikachar, TKV. *Heart of Yoga*. (Rochester, VT: Inner Traditions International, 1995)

———. *Health, Healing, and Beyond*. (New York: Aperture Foundation, Inc., 1998)

Kraftsow, Gary. *Yoga for Wellness*. (New York: Penguin/Arkana, 1999)

———. *Yoga for Transformation*. (New York: Penguin Compass, 2002)

Tibetan Book of Living and Dying (San Francisco: Harper, 2002)

INDEX

Page numbers in *italic* indicate illustrations.

ABOUT THE AUTHOR

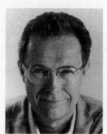

Jeff Davis

Fred Miller is an author and yoga teacher. He has practiced yoga for twenty-four years and has taught yoga for twenty-one. Fred worked in television for twenty-five years in blue and white-collar jobs. Yoga saved his sanity and facilitated a long, successful career in the entertainment industry.

If you have questions or want more information, e-mail *fred@yogafor commonachesandpains.com* or visit his Web site at www.yogaforcommon achesandpains.com.